PALEO SIMPLE

Quarto.com
© 2025 Quarto Publishing Group USA Inc.
Text © 2020 Ashley McCrary
Text © 2020 Christina Shoemaker
Text © 2020 Monica Stevens Le
Text © 2020 Jessica DeMay

First Published in 2025 by Fair Winds Press, an imprint of
The Quarto Group, 100 Cummings Center, Suite 265-D,
Beverly, MA 01915, USA.
T (978) 282-9590 F (978) 283-2742

Fair Winds Press titles are also available at discount for
retail, wholesale, promotional, and bulk purchase. For details,
contact the Special Sales Manager by email at specialsales@
quarto.com or by mail at The Quarto Group, Attn: Special
Sales Manager, 100 Cummings Center, Suite 265-D, Beverly,
MA 01915, USA.

29 28 27 26 25   1 2 3 4 5

ISBN: 978-0-7603-9649-0

Digital edition published in 2025
eISBN: 978-0-7603-9650-6

Library of Congress Cataloging-in-Publication Data available.

The content in this book was previously published in *Clean
Paleo Family Cookbook* by Ashley McCrary (Fair Winds Press,
2020), *Clean Paleo Comfort Food Cookbook* by Jessica DeMay
(Fair Winds Press, 2021), *Clean Paleo One-Pot Meals* by Chris-
tina Shoemaker (Fair Winds Press, 2020), and *Clean Paleo
Real Life* by Monica Stevens Le (Fair Winds Press, 2020).

Design and Page Layout: Kelley Galbreath
Cover images: Ashley McCrary
Photography:
Ashley McCrary: pages 39, 46, 49, 93, 109, 110, 115, 116, 179,
187-191, 201-205, 211

Beth Solano: pages 4, 7

Christina Shoemaker: pages 13, 19, 23, 24, 27, 28, 63-80, 121,
122, 129, 130, 135, 139, 140, 143, 144, 149-155, 213

Meredith Brown: page 57

Monica Stevens Le: pages 8, 11, 41, 45, 59, 95, 97, 98, 101,
105, 181, 182, 199

Joe St. Pierre Photography: pages 36, 35, 50, 54, 85, 86, 91,
159, 160,165-169, 175, 197, 214-228

Printed in China

PALEO SIMPLE

150 DELICIOUS
WHOLE-FOOD MEALS
for HEALTHY LIVING

RECIPES BY
Ashley McCrary, Jessica DeMay,
Christina Shoemaker & Monica Stevens Le

FAIR WINDS

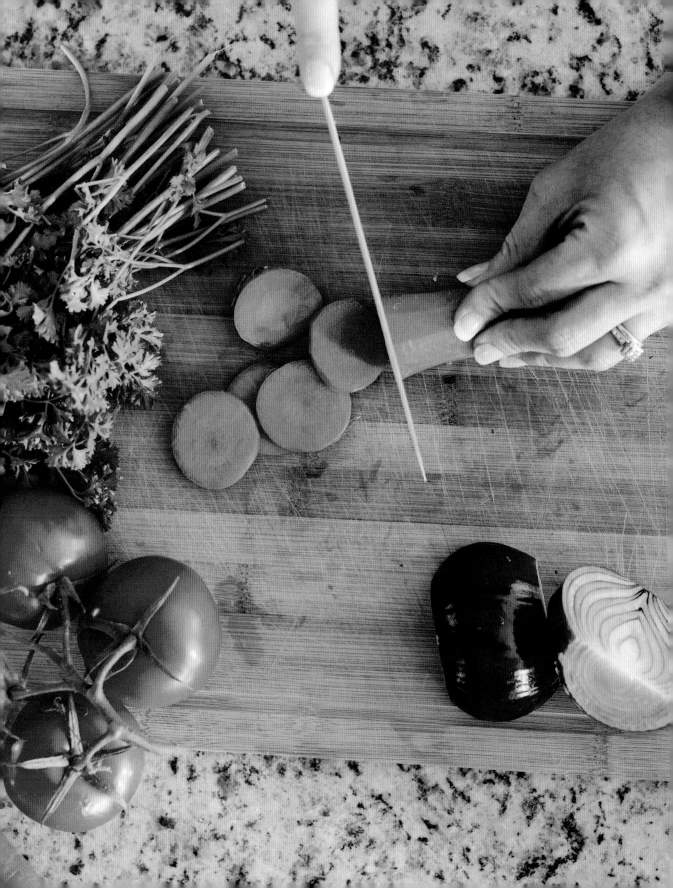

Contents

Introduction

Each of the recipes in this cookbook was designed around the paleo diet. The idea behind paleo eating comes from our hunter-gatherer ancestors and what they ate thousands of years ago. It's based on eating whole, unrefined, and unprocessed foods.

Foods to Eat on the Paleo Diet

- **MEAT:** Beef, lamb, chicken, turkey, pork, and game meats.

- **SEAFOOD:** Salmon, trout, haddock, scallops, shrimp, shellfish, sardines, anchovies, and tuna.

- **EGGS:** Free-range, pastured, or omega-3-enriched eggs.

- **VEGETABLES:** Broccoli, cauliflower, kale, peppers, onions, carrots, radishes, tomatoes, zucchini, squash, salad greens, cucumbers, green beans, snow peas, snap peas, etc.

- **FRUITS:** Apples, bananas, oranges, pears, avocados, berries, melons, and pineapple, etc.

- **TUBERS:** Sweet potatoes, yams, turnips, and beets (but stay away from white potatoes).

- **NUTS AND SEEDS:** Almonds, macadamia nuts, walnuts, hazelnuts, sunflower seeds, pumpkin seeds, pecans, cashews, and flax seeds.

- **HEALTHY FATS AND OILS:** Extra virgin olive oil, light olive oil, coconut oil, avocado oil, sesame oil, and ghee.

- **SPICES:** Sea salt, fresh and dried herbs and spices such as garlic, turmeric, rosemary, basil, oregano, dill, ground mustard seed, paprika, chili powder, and more.

- **FLOURS:** Almond, coconut, cassava, hazelnut, and plantain flours along with arrowroot starch/flour and tapioca starch/flour.

Foods to Avoid on the Paleo Diet

- **SUGAR AND HIGH-FRUCTOSE CORN SYRUP:** Soft drinks, fruit juices, table sugar, candy, pastries, ice cream, and any other form of highly processed and sugary treat.

- **GRAINS:** Breads, pastas, and cereals made with wheat, spelt, rye, barley, oat, rice, and corn.

- **LEGUMES:** Beans (except for green beans), soybeans, chickpeas, peas (except for snow and snap peas), black-eyed peas, peanuts, and lentils.

- **DAIRY:** Avoid dairy, especially low fat (though some versions of paleo do include full-fat dairy like grass-fed ghee).

- **SOME OILS:** Soybean oil, sunflower oil, cottonseed oil, corn oil, grapeseed oil, and safflower oil.

- **TRANS FATS:** Found in margarine and various processed foods. Usually referred to as "hydrogenated" or "partially hydrogenated" oils.

- **ARTIFICIAL SWEETENERS:** Aspartame, sucralose, cyclamates, saccharin, and acesulfame potassium. Use natural sweeteners instead.

- **HIGHLY PROCESSED FOODS:** Anything labeled "diet" or "low fat" or that has many additives.

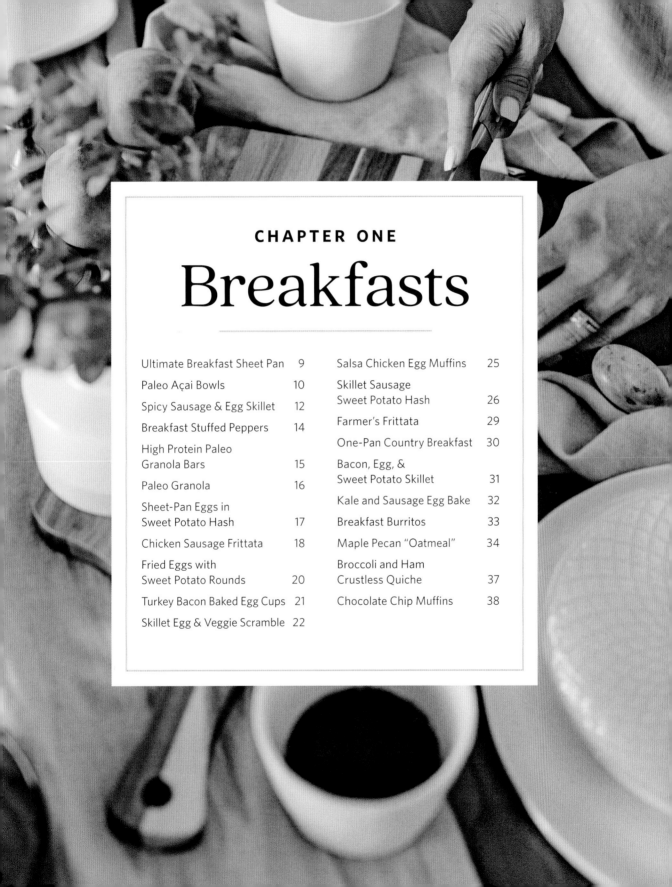

CHAPTER ONE

Breakfasts

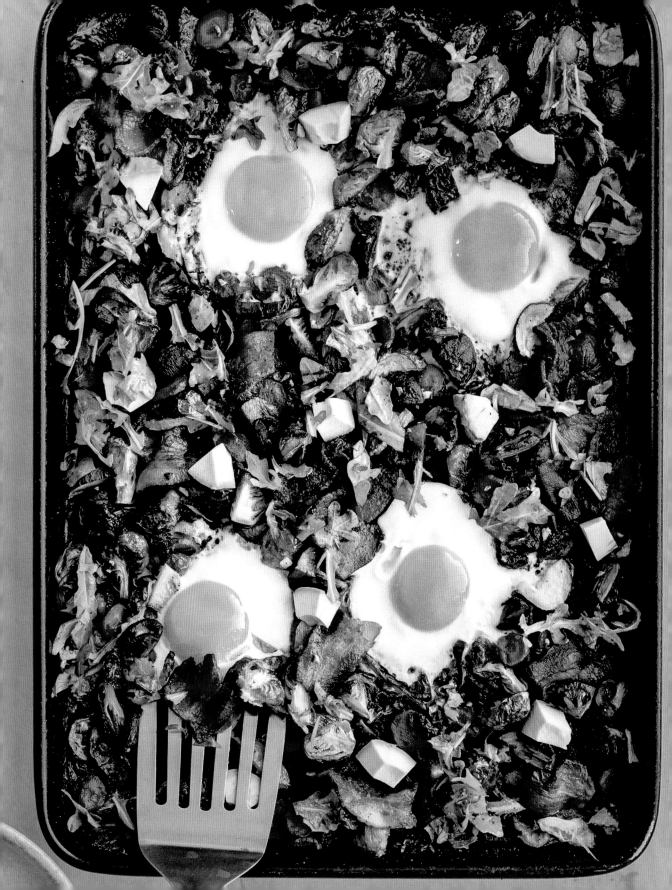

Ultimate Breakfast Sheet Pan

YIELD: 4 SERVINGS

I simply adore how low-maintenance it is to create a one-pan breakfast dish. This is especially true when that breakfast includes bacon, eggs, and all kinds of vegetables that will leave you feeling satisfied (and excited that you ate so many veggies for breakfast!). Get a jump start on it by cutting all the veggies before you go to bed. This breakfast is topped off with diced avocado and fresh herbs, and it's the absolute perfect way to start your morning.

2 tablespoons (30 ml) avocado oil, divided

3 cups (10 ounces or 280 g) Brussels sprouts, trimmed and halved

3 carrots, sliced

1 large zucchini, thinly sliced

1 small yellow onion, sliced

5 ounces (140 g) cremini or baby bella mushrooms, coarsely chopped

Kosher salt, to taste

Black pepper, to taste

6 strips bacon, cut into large chunks

6 cloves garlic, minced

4 large eggs

1 avocado, diced

Chopped fresh parsley (or favorite herb), for garnish

Preheat the oven to 425°F (220°C) and adjust the oven rack to the middle position.

Pour 1 tablespoon (15 ml) of the oil onto a rimmed baking sheet and spread it around evenly using a pastry brush or paper towel.

Arrange the Brussels sprouts, carrots, zucchini, onion, and mushrooms on the baking sheet, but do not overcrowd (use a second sheet pan, if necessary). Drizzle with the remaining 1 tablespoon (15 ml) oil and sprinkle sparingly with salt and pepper (the bacon will add quite a bit of saltiness).

Arrange the bacon over the veggies. Roast for 15 minutes. Remove from the oven and sprinkle the entire pan with the garlic. Give everything a good stir and return the pan to the oven until the veggies are cooked through and the bacon looks crisp, another 15 minutes.

Create four wells for the eggs in the veggies. Carefully crack an egg into a small bowl and pour into a well. (This will ensure you do not break the egg.) Repeat for all the eggs. Return the pan to the oven and bake until the eggs have cooked to your desired level of doneness. (I remove mine after 6 minutes.)

Remove from the oven and serve immediately, topped with the avocado and parsley.

Paleo Açai Bowls

YIELD: 2 BOWLS

These pretty, fruit-filled bowls are packed with all kinds of nutrient-dense ingredients, like creamy cashew butter, coconut oil, and hemp seeds. They're the perfect balance of tart and sweet, and your whole family will love them. I like to play around with toppings, using strawberries, blueberries, bananas, cacao nibs, and bee pollen. What a refreshing way to start the day!

1 packet (3.5 ounces [70 g]) frozen, unsweetened açai (see Notes)

1¼ cups (225 g) frozen mixed berries

1 small frozen banana

½ cup (120 ml) unsweetened coconut or almond milk (see Notes)

2 tablespoons (22 g) hemp seeds or chia seeds

2 scoops collagen peptides (omit for vegan, see Notes)

1 heaping tablespoon (15 g) cashew butter or almond butter

1 tablespoon (15 ml) coconut oil

Toppings of choice (see headnote for ideas)

In the pitcher of a high-speed blender, add the açai, berries, banana, milk, seeds, collagen (if using), nut butter, and coconut oil.

Blend on medium-high speed for 1 minute. Scrape the sides or use the tamper to make sure everything gets blended well.

Pour into two bowls and top with your favorite toppings.

Notes

The açai comes already pureed and frozen in individual-serving-size packages.

This recipe uses coconut milk from a carton, not the canned variety.

If you are omitting the collagen peptides, be sure to make up the thickness by using an extra ¼ to ⅓ cup (40 to 50 g) frozen berries.

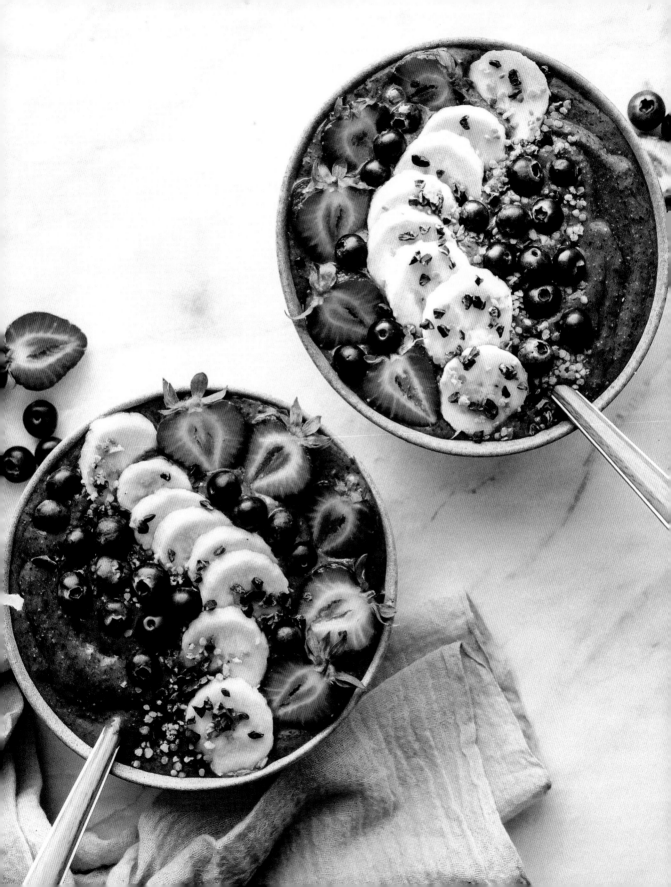

Spicy Sausage & Egg Skillet

YIELD: 4 SERVINGS

Use your favorite precooked sausage to create a flavorful egg scramble that packs some heat! Amp up the intensity with extra hot sauce in the eggs and a hefty dose of sriracha before serving.

3 tablespoons (42 g) ghee, divided (see Note)

1 cup (70 g) sliced mushrooms

2 precooked sausages, sliced ¼-inch (6 mm) thick

1 teaspoon minced garlic

8 large eggs

1½ teaspoons hot sauce (see Note)

¾ teaspoon salt

¼ teaspoon chipotle chile powder

Sriracha sauce

Add 2 tablespoons (28 g) of the ghee, the mushrooms, and the sausage to a large skillet over medium-high heat. Sauté until the mushrooms are soft and the sausage has some browning, 3 to 4 minutes. Add the garlic. Stir and give it a quick sauté, about 1 minute, to achieve a golden color.

Meanwhile, whisk together the eggs, ¼ cup (60 ml) water, hot sauce, salt, and chile powder in a medium bowl. (The water helps make the eggs a little more fluffy since we're not using milk.)

Reduce the heat to medium-low. Add the remaining 1 tablespoon (14 g) ghee to the skillet. Pour the egg mixture over the mushroom mixture. The eggs will begin cooking right away. Use a spatula to fold the cooked outer edges of the eggs toward the center. Do this repeatedly until you don't have any more liquid in the pan.

Serve topped with a hearty drizzle of your favorite sriracha sauce.

Notes

You can easily substitute a different cooking fat for ghee if you're completely dairy free or just prefer an alternative. I use ghee because it's my absolute favorite for eggs!

Check out the ingredients in your hot sauce and sriracha sauce.

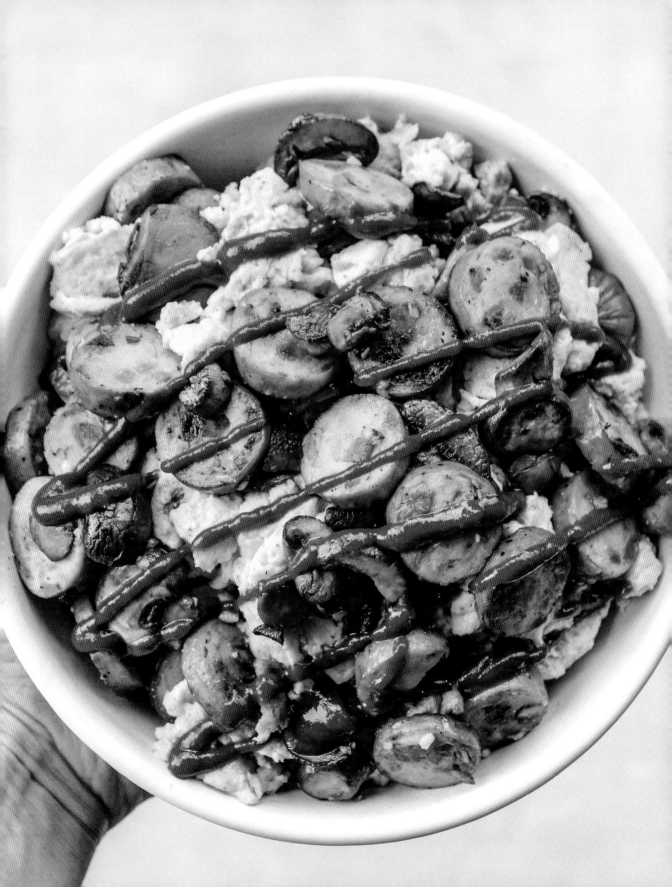

Breakfast Stuffed Peppers

YIELD: 6 PEPPERS

Stuffed peppers aren't just for dinner, especially when the savory ground beef is mixed with fluffy scrambled eggs. I add my own special touch with a drizzle of homemade avocado-ranch.

3 multicolor bell peppers, halved and seeded

1 tablespoon (15 ml) olive oil

1 clove garlic, minced

1 pound (454 g) 90 / 10 ground beef

6 large eggs

2 tablespoons (30 ml) canned unsweetened coconut milk

2 tablespoons (8 g) nutritional yeast

1 tablespoon (15 ml) lime juice

½ teaspoon sea salt

¼ teaspoon black pepper

1 cup paleo-friendly ranch dressing

1 small avocado, peeled and pitted

Fresh coarsely chopped parsley or cilantro, for garnish

Preheat the oven to 400°F (200°C or gas mark 6) and grease a baking sheet with olive oil.

Place the peppers cut-side up on the baking sheet. Bake until tender, about 20 minutes.

Meanwhile, heat the olive oil and garlic in a large skillet over medium-high heat.

Add the ground beef and use a wooden spoon to break it up. Cook until brown and no longer pink, 6 to 7 minutes.

Pour the beef into a bowl and set aside.

In a medium bowl, whisk together the eggs, coconut milk, nutritional yeast, lime juice, salt, and pepper.

Pour the egg mixture into the skillet and reduce the heat to low. Using a wooden spoon or spatula, move the eggs back and forth and cook until fluffy, about 5 minutes.

Add back the cooked ground beef and fold together with the spoon until combined.

Remove the peppers from the oven and fill each with the egg-beef mixture.

Return the peppers to the oven and bake for 10 minutes more.

Meanwhile, in a wide-mouth mason jar or small bowl, add the ranch and avocado. Using an immersion blender, blend together until creamy. (You may also do this in a regular blender.)

Allow the peppers to cool slightly before plating, drizzled with the avocado-ranch and topped with parsley.

If there is dressing left, add to a mason jar and cap with a lid. Will keep in the refrigerator for a day or two. Due to the nature of the avocado, it may turn brown if stored any longer.

High Protein Paleo Granola Bars

YIELD: 8 BARS

What if I told you that in 10 minutes you could make homemade paleo granola bars that are as nutritious as they are delicious? This awesome mixture of nuts and seeds tastes fabulous with cacao nibs, creamy cashew butter, and raisins. Feel free to get creative and swap out some of the nuts or seeds for your favorites. These bars are perfect with breakfast, as a snack, or to grab and go, go, go!

½ cup (75 g) raw cashews

½ cup (75 g) walnuts

½ cup (75 g) pumpkin seeds

⅓ cup (50 g) unsweet- ened raisins

5 tablespoons (30 g) collagen peptides

3 tablespoons (33 g) chia seeds

3 tablespoons (36 g) flaxseeds

2 tablespoons (15 g) cacao nibs

½ cup (120 g) creamy cashew butter

3 tablespoons (45 ml) coconut oil

2 tablespoons (30 ml) pure maple syrup

1 teaspoon (5 ml) pure vanilla extract

Line an 8 x 8-inch (20.5 x 20.5 cm) baking dish with parchment paper.

In the bowl of a food processor, add the cashews, walnuts, pumpkin seeds, raisins, collagen, chia, flax, and cacao nibs. Pulse several times until coarse throughout. Transfer the mixture to a large bowl and set aside.

In a small saucepan, combine the cashew butter, coconut oil, syrup, and vanilla over low heat. Mix thoroughly until smooth and creamy through- out, about 1 minute.

Add the wet ingredients to the dry and give everything a good stir.

Transfer the mixture to the prepared baking dish. Press down with the bottom of a glass, jar, or your fingertips to pack it into the bottom of the dish, creating an even base. If it's too sticky, lightly wet your fingertips.

Place in the refrigerator to set overnight. Cut into 8 bars with a sharp knife. Store in an airtight container in the refrigerator for up to 10 days.

Note

Get creative with the nuts and seeds. Feel free to use almonds, pecans, sunflower seeds, etc.

Paleo Granola

Store-bought granolas can be very non-paleo friendly. They're also expensive! My version uses a variety of nuts infused with cinnamon and honey, baked until crispy golden brown, and it's so simple to make. Eat it as a snack or add almond milk to make the perfect paleo cereal.

½ cup (60 g) chopped pecans

½ cup (60 g) chopped walnuts

½ cup (55 g) sliced almonds

½ cup (40 g) unsweetened coconut flakes

⅓ cup (45 g) raw cashew halves

¼ cup (37 g) unsweetened raisins, dried blueberries, or cranberries

1 teaspoon ground cinnamon

½ teaspoon sea salt

½ cup (170 g) raw honey

¼ cup (60 g) coconut oil

1 teaspoon pure vanilla extract

Preheat the oven to 300°F (150°C or gas mark 2) and line a large baking sheet with parchment paper.

In a large bowl, combine the pecans, walnuts, almonds, coconut flakes, cashews, dried fruit, cinnamon, and salt.

In a glass measuring cup, add the honey, coconut oil, and vanilla. Heat in the microwave for 30 seconds. Stir to combine.

Pour the warm liquid over the nut mixture and stir together until everything is well combined and coated.

Spread the mixture evenly on the prepared baking sheet. Bake until it is golden and crispy, about 20 minutes.

Remove from the oven and let cool on the baking sheet for 10 minutes.

Break the granola with your hands or a fork.

Cool completely and store in an airtight container in a dry place for up to 6 months.

Note

You can freeze granola, wrapped tightly in plastic wrap and/or in a resealable freezer bag.

Sheet-Pan Eggs in Sweet Potato Hash

YIELD: 4 SERVINGS

Keep breakfast simple with a tasty hash of sweet potato, onion, and baked eggs. You'll only need a few ingredients!

2 large sweet potatoes, cut into ½-inch (1 cm) cubes

½ large white or yellow onion, diced into ½-inch (1 cm) pieces

1½ teaspoons extra-virgin olive oil or coconut oil

4 large eggs

Salt

Handful of fresh herbs, chopped (basil, cilantro, or parsley work great)

Preheat the oven to 425°F (220°C, or gas mark 7).

Spread the sweet potatoes and onion in a single layer on a 9½ x 13-inch (24 x 33 cm) baking sheet. (This is a quarter sheet pan. While I typically recommend a 12 x 17-inch [30 x 43 cm] pan for most sheet-pan meals, the ingredients for this recipe won't take up much space, so a quarter pan is perfect.)

Drizzle the oil over the veggies. Give it all a quick stir. Spread in an even layer.

Bake for 15 minutes. Remove from the oven and stir. Spread again in an even layer.

Use a spatula to create four little spaces for your eggs. Crack one egg into each hole. Sprinkle salt on the eggs. Bake until the egg whites are set and the egg yolks are cooked to how you like them, 5 to 8 minutes.

Remove from the oven and sprinkle fresh herbs on top before serving.

Chicken Sausage Frittata

YIELD: 8 SLICES

This fully loaded frittata is inspired by my all-time favorite breakfast casserole by a similar name, but it cooks even faster. It's packed with flavor thanks to the salsa whisked into the eggs, and the chicken sausage, spinach, and riced sweet potato.

2 tablespoons (28 ml) extra-virgin olive oil or (28 g) ghee (For dairy-free dishes, use extra-virgin olive oil.)

½ white or yellow onion, diced into ½-inch (1 cm) pieces

1 cup (about 5 ounces, or 140 g) riced or shredded sweet potato (see Note)

9 large eggs

½ cup (130 g) salsa

½ teaspoon salt

½ teaspoon black pepper

1 packed cup (about half a 5-ounce, or 140 g, package) baby spinach

2 fully cooked chicken sausages, sliced ¼-inch (6 mm) thick (see Note)

Preheat the oven to 425°F (220°C, or gas mark 7).

Add the oil or ghee, onion, and sweet potato to a cast-iron skillet over medium-high heat. Sauté until the onion is softened and the potato has some browning, stirring frequently, 3 to 5 minutes.

Meanwhile, whisk together the eggs, salsa, salt, and black pepper in a large bowl. Set aside.

When the onion is done, turn off the stove. Spread the onion and potato mixture across the bottom of the skillet so it is evenly distributed. Layer the spinach leaves on top and then layer on your chicken sausage. Pour your egg mixture over everything.

Bake until the center is just set, 18 to 20 minutes. Check to make sure the center isn't very wiggly and then remove from the oven. Let it rest for a few minutes before serving.

Notes

I use chicken sausage that's gluten and casein free and has no added nitrates. Use whatever brand you like or even swap it out for beef or turkey sausage!

I use frozen riced sweet potato. The only ingredient is sweet potato. I don't even thaw it before sautéing! You can also shred or rice your own sweet potato at home if you prefer.

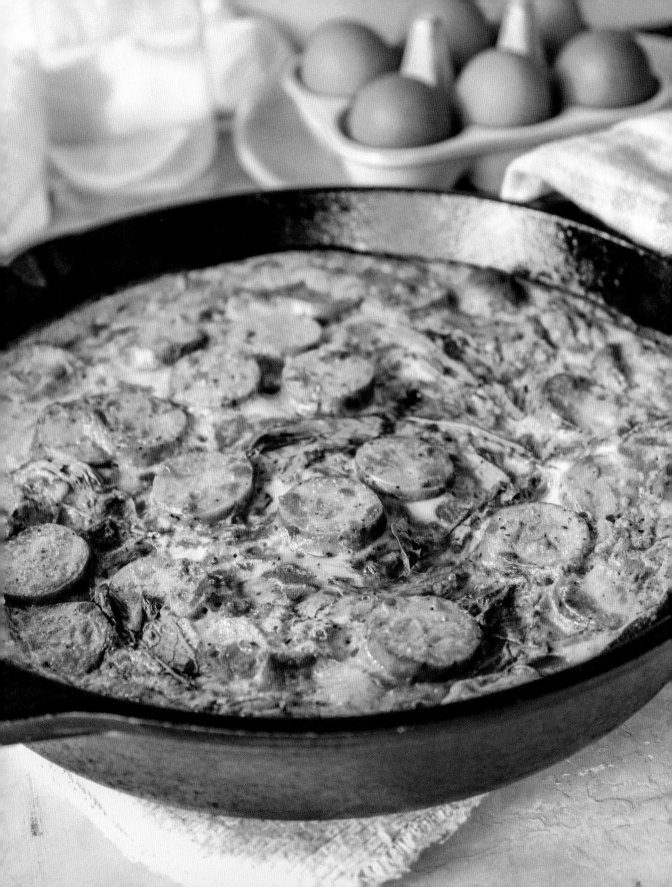

Fried Eggs with Sweet Potato Rounds

YIELD: 2 SERVINGS

Sometimes, you don't need anything more than eggs and potatoes. This whole dish cooks in less than 15 minutes. It's perfect for two!

1 medium sweet potato, cut into ¼-inch (6 mm)-thick rounds

½ teaspoon salt, plus more to taste

½ teaspoon paprika

2 tablespoons (28 g) coconut oil

1 tablespoon (15 g) ghee (see Note)

2 to 4 large eggs

Black pepper, to taste

In a large bowl, toss your potato rounds in the salt and paprika so they're well seasoned.

Add the oil to a large nonstick skillet over medium-high heat. Once hot, add half of the potato rounds. You should hear a sizzle when you add them to the skillet. Cook for 2½ to 4 minutes until the side touching the skillet has some browning. Flip and cook for another 2½ to 4 minutes. Remove the rounds from the skillet and place on a paper towel–lined plate.

Repeat with the remaining potato rounds. If you're low on oil, add another ½ tablespoon before doing the second half. All the potato rounds should be on the plate when finished.

Reduce the heat to medium and wipe out the skillet.

Add the ghee to the cleaned skillet. Once melted, crack the eggs on one side of the skillet and sprinkle with salt and black pepper. Place the potato rounds beside the eggs. Cover the skillet and cook until the egg whites are set and the egg yolks are cooked to how you like them, about 3 minutes.

Note

You can easily substitute a different cooking fat for ghee if you're completely dairy free or just prefer an alternative. I use ghee because it's my absolute favorite for eggs!

Turkey Bacon Baked Egg Cups

YIELD: 12 EGG CUPS

Eggs and bacon are the two most essential breakfast items of all the essential breakfast items. Am I right? I'm right. So, let's bake them together! If you're new to cooking with turkey bacon, you'll quickly discover that there are some fantastic brands and some less fantastic brands. I really recommend the thick, minimally processed turkey bacon you'll find in the natural foods section of your grocery store. It's so much more delicious, it's better for you, and it will better replicate that pork bacon we all grew up loving.

1½ to 2 tablespoons (23 to 28 ml) extra-virgin olive oil

12 slices turkey bacon, halved crosswise

12 large eggs

Salt and black pepper

Preheat the oven to 400°F (200°C, or gas mark 6). Grease a 12-cup muffin tin with oil, making sure you cover both the sides and the bottom of each cup. Wipe up any excess oil so you don't have oil pooling in the bottom of the cups.

Crisscross 2 bacon halves in the bottom of each cup to create an X.

Bake for 10 to 12 minutes. If the bacon you're using is thick (you did buy the better bacon, didn't you?), bake for 12 minutes. If you're using a fairly thin bacon (typically what's available in most supermarkets), 10 minutes will be fine. Your bacon will not be quite done.

Remove from the oven and carefully crack an egg on top of the bacon in each cup. Sprinkle with salt and black pepper.

Place back in the oven for 10 minutes or until the egg whites are set and the egg yolks are cooked to how you like them. Serve immediately!

Skillet Egg & Veggie Scramble

Are you tired of boring eggs? Well, this scramble will change your mind! Salsa and sautéed veggies make these eggs next-level good. You'll never want to make plain scrambled eggs again.

2 tablespoons (28 g) ghee, divided

1 cup (71 g) chopped broccoli florets

½ white or yellow onion, diced into ½-inch (1 cm) pieces

8 large eggs

¼ cup (65 g) salsa

½ teaspoon salt

¼ teaspoon black pepper

1 packed cup (about half a 5-ounce, or 140 g, package) baby spinach

½ cup (90 g) halved grape tomatoes

Add 1 tablespoon (14 g) of the ghee to a large skillet over medium-high heat. Once hot, add the broccoli and onion. Sauté, stirring occasionally, until the onion is tender and you see some browning on the broccoli, 3 to 5 minutes.

Meanwhile, whisk together the eggs, salsa, salt, and black pepper in a bowl. Set aside.

When the onions and broccoli are done, reduce the heat to medium or medium-low. Add the remaining 1 tablespoon (14 g) ghee to the skillet. Pour in the egg mixture, spinach, and tomatoes. Use a spatula to fold the cooked outer edges of the eggs toward the center. Do this repeatedly until you don't have any more liquid in the skillet.

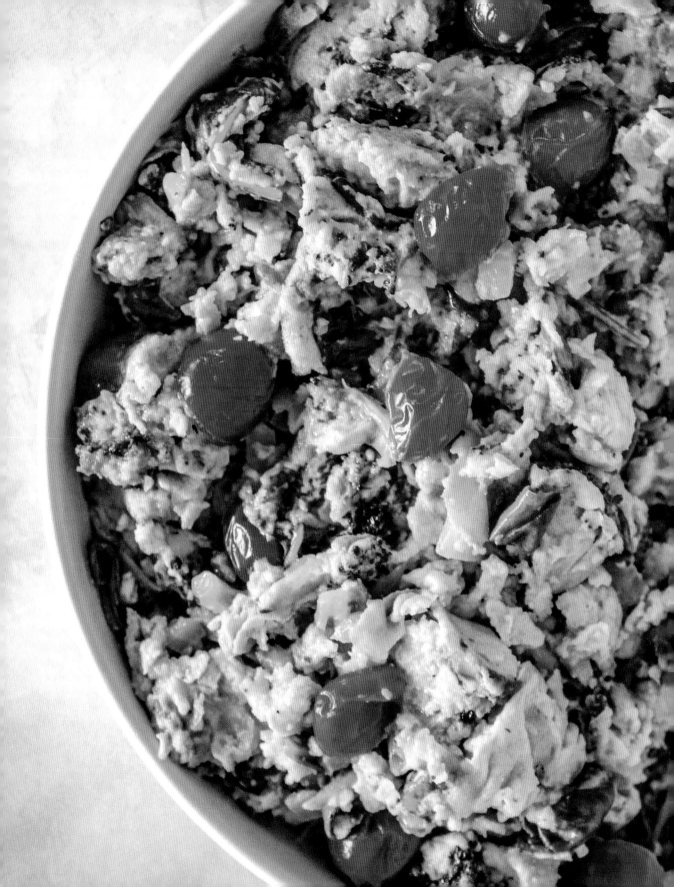

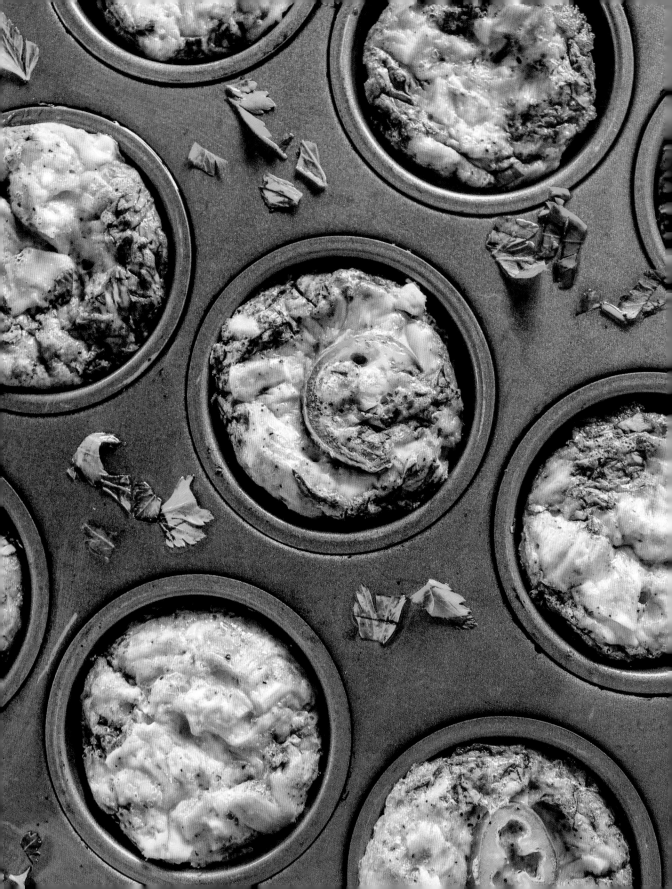

Salsa Chicken Egg Muffins

YIELD: 12 MUFFINS

These savory muffins are perfect for meal prep or for when you want a healthy breakfast option for a crowd. Serve them with extra salsa or even guacamole. Or, keep them stocked in the fridge for a grab-and-go breakfast!

1½ tablespoons (25 ml) extra-virgin olive oil

12 large eggs

½ cup (130 g) salsa

½ teaspoon salt

½ teaspoon black pepper

¼ cup (8 g) chopped fresh spinach

¾ cup (94 g) shredded cooked chicken (see Note)

Fresh jalapeño slices (optional)

Preheat the oven to 350°F (180°C, or gas mark 4). Grease a 12-cup muffin tin with the oil. Don't skimp on this or your eggs will stick. Make sure you grease both the sides and the bottom of each muffin cup.

In a large bowl, whisk together the eggs with the salsa, salt, and black pepper.

Pour the egg mixture evenly into each cup, so they're about three-fourths of the way full (or a little more).

Divide the spinach among each cup and use a fork to push the spinach down a bit. Divide the chicken among the cups. Add a slice of jalapeño to the top of your muffins, if using. (I do this for half of my egg muffins so that I have six that are spicy and six that aren't.)

Bake until the eggs are puffed and just set, about 20 minutes. Remove from the oven and set aside to cool. The egg muffins will puff up a lot while baking but will settle down over the next 5 minutes as they cool. Once cooled, use a fork or small spatula to gently pull the egg muffins from the pan.

Notes

Purchase a rotisserie chicken from your grocery store to save time.

Try these optional additions: diced onion, diced bell pepper, or fresh cilantro.

To reheat muffins, microwave each for around 15 seconds, adding more time, if necessary.

To freeze, pop completely cooled muffins into a resealable plastic bag and place them in the freezer. When you're ready to reheat, wrap each muffin in a wet paper towel (to help hold in the moisture) and heat in the microwave for about 30 seconds, adding more time, if necessary.

Skillet Sausage Sweet Potato Hash

YIELD: 4 SERVINGS

This simple hash has plenty of flavor and comes together in 25 minutes!

2 tablespoons (28 ml) extra-virgin olive oil or cooking fat of choice

2 cups (266 g) diced sweet potatoes, ½-inch (1 cm) cubes

¼ white or yellow onion, diced into ½-inch (1 cm) pieces

1 teaspoon salt, divided, plus more to taste

¼ teaspoon paprika

½ pound (225 g) ground turkey or pork sausage

½ teaspoon chili powder

½ teaspoon dried oregano

¼ teaspoon garlic powder

¼ teaspoon black pepper, plus more to taste

4 large eggs

Add the oil to a large skillet over medium-high heat. Once hot, add the potatoes and onion. Sauté, stirring occasionally, until the potatoes have browned and the onion is tender, about 5 minutes. Stir in ½ teaspoon of the salt and the paprika. Remove from the skillet and set aside.

Crumble the ground meat into the skillet and return to medium-high heat. Sauté until browned and cooked through, about 7 minutes. Stir in the remaining ½ teaspoon salt, chili powder, oregano, garlic powder, and black pepper.

Add the potatoes and onions back to the skillet. Use your spatula to create four holes in the hash. Crack one egg into each hole and sprinkle with salt and pepper. Cover the skillet and reduce the heat to medium. Cook until the egg whites are set and the yolks are cooked to how you like them, 5 to 8 minutes.

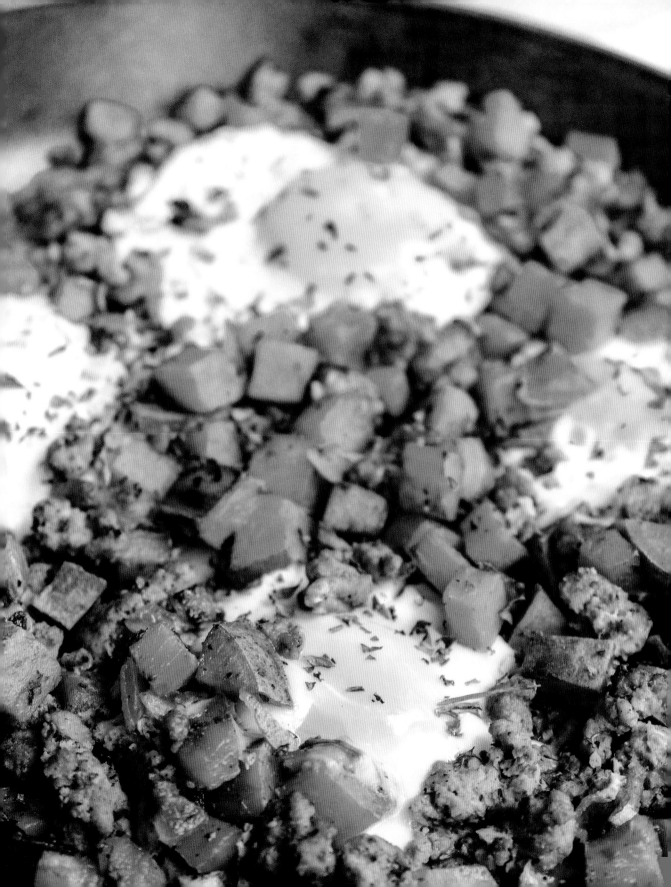

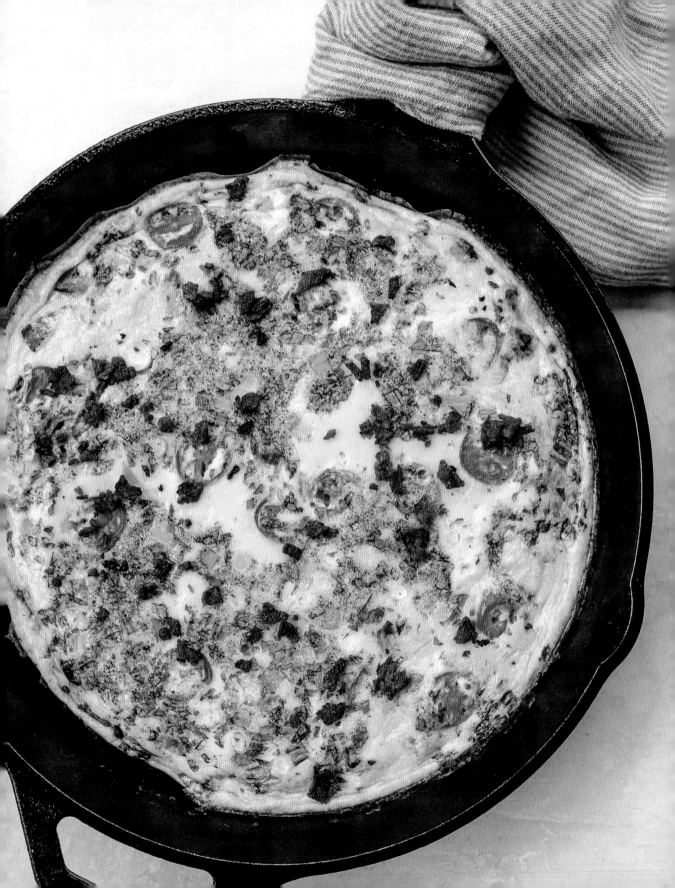

Farmer's Frittata

YIELD: 8 SLICES

Frittatas are one of my favorite ways to celebrate breakfast because there are so many ways to mix up the flavors! Plus, they always look extra special so guests think you've been working hard in the kitchen. There's no need to tell them how easy this frittata is to throw together. It will be our secret.

1 cup (133 g) diced sweet potatoes, ½-inch (1 cm) cubes

5 slices bacon (turkey or pork), diced

¼ white or yellow onion, diced into ½-inch (1 cm) pieces

9 large eggs

1 teaspoon salt

½ teaspoon black pepper

¼ teaspoon ground mustard

½ cup (75 g) cherry or (90 g) grape tomatoes, halved

2 scallions, thinly sliced

2 tablespoons (8 g) chopped fresh parsley

Preheat the oven to 425°F (220°C, or gas mark 7).

Add the sweet potatoes, bacon, and onion to a large cast-iron skillet over medium-high heat. Sauté until the veggies are softened, about 5 minutes. (If using turkey bacon, add 2 tablespoons [28 ml] cooking fat to the skillet.)

Meanwhile, in a large bowl, whisk together the eggs, ½ cup (120 ml) water, salt, black pepper, and mustard.

Turn off the stove. Spread the sweet potato mixture across the bottom of the skillet so it's evenly distributed. Pour in the egg mixture. Sprinkle the tomatoes, scallions, and parsley on top.

Bake until just set, 10 to 12 minutes. Check to make sure the center isn't wiggly and then remove from the oven. Let your frittata rest for 5 minutes before serving.

Note

Cast iron is a naturally nonstick surface, so if it's been seasoned correctly, food won't stick. However, if your cast iron isn't well cared for, then sticking may be an issue. If you're concerned about the state of your skillet, wipe it down with olive oil before using it for this frittata recipe. After each use, wipe the inside of your skillet with a very thin layer of olive oil, just enough that the skillet is glossy. You don't want any oil to pool and settle when you put the skillet away or it will get sticky. You'll soon start to love your cast-iron skillet again!

One-Pan Country Breakfast

YIELD: 4 SERVINGS

When you order a country breakfast in a restaurant, you'll usually receive a plate of cheesy eggs, potatoes with bell peppers, and ham or bacon. My spin on it is better for you but still ridiculously tasty. We're keeping it low carb with butternut squash, and it's dairy free, of course.

2 tablespoons (28 ml) extra-virgin olive oil, divided

1 red bell pepper, diced into ½-inch (1 cm) pieces

½ white or yellow onion, diced into ½-inch (1 cm) pieces

1 cup (140 g) diced butternut squash, ¾ to 1 inch (2 to 2.5 cm) cubes (see Notes)

1 cup chopped cooked (140 g) turkey, (150 g) ham, or (140 g) chicken

8 large eggs

½ teaspoon salt

¼ teaspoon black pepper

Add 1 tablespoon (15 ml) of the olive oil to a large skillet over medium-high heat. Once hot, add the bell pepper and onion. Sauté, stirring occasionally, for 2 minutes. (They won't be quite finished yet.) Add the squash and cooked protein. Sauté everything until the squash is tender, the onion is softened, and the bell pepper has some browning, 3 to 5 minutes.

Meanwhile, in a medium bowl, whisk together the eggs, ¼ cup (60 ml) water, salt, and black pepper. Set aside.

Reduce the heat to medium or medium-low. Add the remaining 1 tablespoon (15 ml) oil to the skillet. Pour the eggs over the squash mixture. Use a spatula to fold the cooked outer edges of the eggs toward the center. Do this repeatedly until you don't have any more liquid in the pan.

Notes

Cut the butternut squash into cubes ¾ to 1 inch (2 to 2.5 cm) big. Some grocery stores carry prechopped squash in this very size. It's a huge time-saver!

This is a great recipe for using leftover Thanksgiving turkey, rotisserie chicken, or holiday ham. Deli meat works well here, too.

Bacon, Egg & Sweet Potato Skillet

YIELD: 4 SERVINGS

If you don't have any experience making a hash, this is the perfect recipe to start with! And who doesn't enjoy bacon, eggs, and potatoes? This uncomplicated breakfast skillet wins everybody over and is ready in about 15 minutes.

2 tablespoons (28 ml) extra-virgin olive oil or cooking fat of choice

4 cups (532 g) diced sweet potatoes, ½-inch (1 cm) cubes

4 slices bacon (turkey or pork), chopped (see Note)

½ teaspoon salt, plus more to taste

½ teaspoon black pepper, plus more to taste

½ teaspoon paprika

4 large eggs

3 scallions, sliced

Add the oil to a large skillet over medium-high heat. Once hot, add the potatoes and bacon. Sauté, stirring occasionally, until the potatoes have browned, about 5 minutes. The potatoes won't be completely cooked through at this point. We just want them to have some color and crispy edges. Add the salt, black pepper, and paprika, stirring to combine.

Use your spatula to create four holes in the hash. Crack one egg into each hole. Sprinkle with salt and black pepper. Cover the skillet and reduce the heat to medium. Cook until the egg whites are set and the egg yolks are cooked to how you like them, 5 to 8 minutes. Sprinkle with the scallions before serving.

Note

We're using chopped bacon here (not crumbled) so it's substantial enough to hold up to the sweet potatoes but also small enough to cook quickly.

Kale and Sausage Egg Bake

YIELD: 6–8 SERVINGS

You can never have too many breakfast bake ideas! The sweet potato, sausage, and kale bake is hearty and nourishing.

PALEO SIMPLE

1 pound (454 g) sweet potatoes, chopped into ½-inch (1 cm) chunks

2 tablespoons (30 ml) avocado oil, divided

½ teaspoon salt, divided

1 pound (454 g) breakfast sausage, homemade or sugar-free store-bought

5 ounces (142 g) baby kale

12 large eggs

Preheat the oven to 425°F (220°C or gas mark 7). Line a baking sheet with parchment paper. Line a 13 by 9-inch (33 by 23 cm) pan with parchment paper.

Place the sweet potatoes on the prepared baking sheet and toss with 1 tablespoon (15 ml) of the oil and ¼ teaspoon of the salt. Roast for 20 minutes, or until the potatoes are tender.

While the potatoes are cooking, cook the sausage in a large skillet over medium heat for 5–7 minutes, or until cooked through. Place the sausage in the prepared pan, spreading evenly.

Add the remaining 1 tablespoon (15 ml) oil to the skillet used for the sausage and add the kale. Sprinkle with the remaining ¼ teaspoon salt and cook for 2–3 minutes, or until tender. Spread the kale evenly over the sausage.

When the sweet potatoes are done roasting, place them in the pan with the kale and sausage and stir to combine. Reduce the oven temperature to 350°F (180°C or gas mark 4).

Crack the eggs into a medium-size bowl and whisk until well combined. Pour the eggs over the meat mixture. Stir a little if necessary, distributing the ingredients as evenly as possible.

Bake for 45–50 minutes, or until the middle is set. Serve warm.

Store leftovers, covered, in the refrigerator for up to 6 days.

Breakfast Burritos

YIELD: 8 BURRITOS

The dad of one of my high school friends made the best breakfast burritos and I always looked forward to them. Packed with all the fillings and so satisfying, these are a grain-free version, made with almond flour tortillas, but still just as delicious and comforting. They are pretty forgiving if you want to switch up the ingredients, just keep the measurements the same—and play around with your favorite fillings.

8 grain-free tortillas, such as Siete Almond Flour Tortillas

8 pieces sugar-free bacon

½ cup (75 g) diced red bell pepper, about half a large pepper

½ cup (80 g) diced onion, about half a medium onion

¼ teaspoon salt

2 tablespoons (30 ml) ghee

8 large eggs

¼ cup (60 ml) almond milk

¼ teaspoon salt

¼ teaspoon black pepper

Cut bacon and cook in a large skillet over medium heat, stirring regularly, until crispy. About 10 minutes. Turn the heat off and remove from the pan and place on a plate.

Leave the bacon fat in the pan and add in the red pepper and onion. Turn heat back to medium and cook 5 minutes, until softened. Turn off the heat and remove the mixture to a bowl. Wipe down the pan and add the ghee.

In a large bowl, whisk together the eggs and almond milk. Turn the heat to medium and let the ghee melt. Add in the eggs and stir with a rubber spatula until fully cooked through, about 4 minutes. Add in the salt and pepper and mix well. Remove to a small bowl.

Assemble the burritos. Warm the tortillas so they are easy to fold. Baking them for 3 minutes in a 300°F (150°C or gas mark 2) oven works great.

Spread some eggs (about ¼ cup [55 g]) on the bottom, top with peppers and onion then top with the bacon. Fold to close. Repeat with the remaining.

Serve immediately or store in the fridge. Wrap in foil or wax paper to hold together.

Maple Pecan "Oatmeal"

YIELD: 4–6 SERVINGS

You will not miss oatmeal if you have this grain-free version! The coconut and pecans mimic the texture of oatmeal, and the flavor is incredible. This makes a great breakfast or dessert.

2 tablespoons (15 g) coconut flour

1 cup (80 g) unsweetened shredded coconut

1 cup (112 g) raw pecans

1 large egg

⅓ cup (80 ml) maple syrup

1 teaspoon ground cinnamon

½ teaspoon salt

¾ cup (180 ml) almond milk

2 tablespoons (30 ml) melted ghee

Preheat the oven to 325°F (170°C or gas mark 3). Line a 9 by 9-inch (23 by 23 cm) pan with parchment paper.

Combine the coconut flour, shredded coconut, and pecans in a food processor and process for less than 1 minute, or until the mixture is crumbly and all the pieces are similar in size.

Pour the mixture into a large bowl. Add the egg, maple syrup, cinnamon, salt, almond milk, and ghee. Mix well.

Scoop the mixture into the prepared pan and spread evenly. Bake for 35–40 minutes, or until the edges are lightly brown. Cut into slices and serve warm. Add a drizzle of maple syrup and a few fresh berries on top if desired.

Store leftovers, covered, in the refrigerator for up to a week.

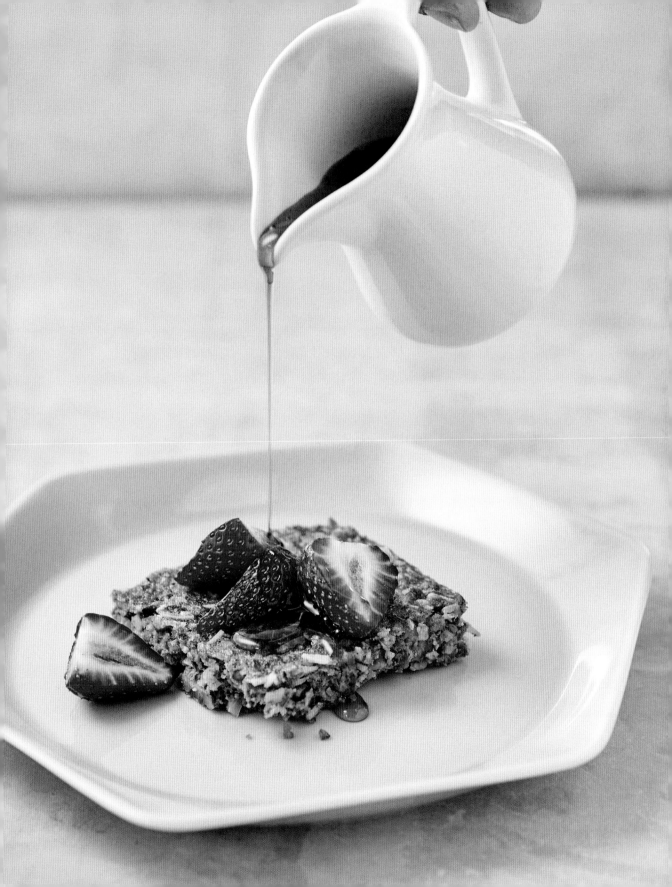

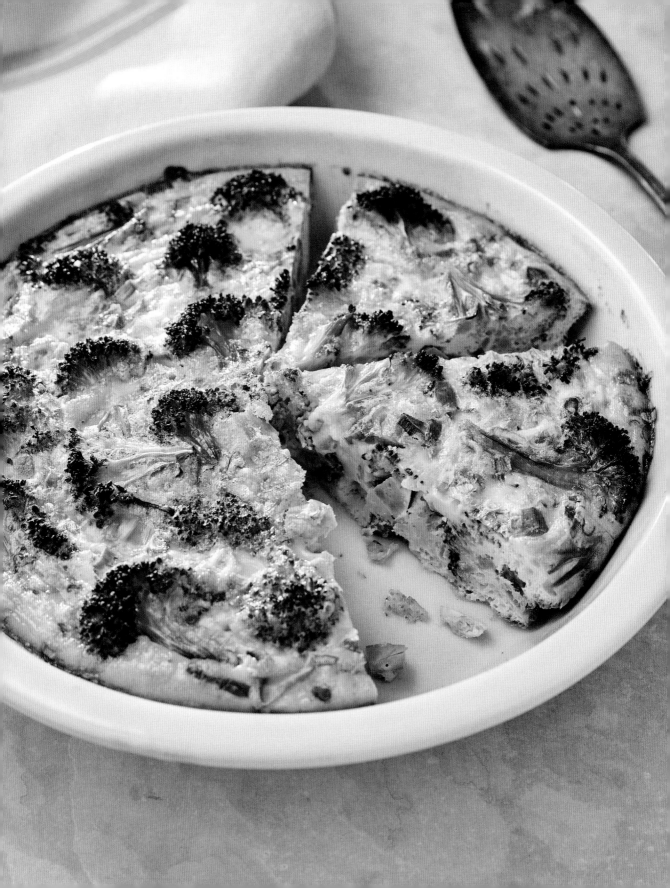

Broccoli and Ham Crustless Quiche

YIELD: 4–6 SERVINGS

A few simple ingredients come together in this recipe to create a pleasing breakfast. This is great served with a side of fruit to make a complete meal.

12 ounces (340 g) frozen broccoli

1 tablespoon (15 ml) avocado oil

10 ounces (283 g) nitrate-free ham, chopped

¼ cup (24 g) chopped green onion

10 eggs

¼ cup (60 ml) almond milk

Preheat the oven to 425°F (220°C or gas mark 7). Line a baking sheet with parchment paper. Grease a deep-dish pie plate well with coconut oil or line it with parchment paper.

Place the broccoli on the prepared baking sheet, drizzle with the avocado oil, and bake for 25 minutes, or until tender.

Place the ham and green onion in the prepared pie dish.

When the broccoli is done roasting, lower the oven temperature to 350°F (180°C or gas mark 4). Spread the broccoli evenly in the pie plate.

Combine the eggs and almond milk in a medium-size bowl. Stir until well mixed, with all the yolks broken. Pour the eggs over the ham mixture. Stir to make sure all the ingredients are distributed evenly.

Bake for 45–50 minutes, or until the center is set. Cut into slices and serve warm.

Store leftovers, covered, in the refrigerator for up to 6 days.

Chocolate Chip Muffins

YIELD: 10 MUFFINS

These muffins are soft, moist, and loaded with chocolate chips. They are super easy to make with just a handful of ingredients, and they're a treat the whole family will love.

2 cups (224 g) almond flour

¼ cup (30 g) coconut flour

½ teaspoon baking soda

¼ teaspoon salt

⅓ cup (80 ml) maple syrup or honey

¼ cup (60 ml) melted ghee

3 large eggs, at room temperature

½ cup (85 g) dairy-free chocolate chips

Preheat the oven to 350°F (180°C or gas mark 4). Line a muffin pan with 10 parchment liners.

Combine the almond flour, coconut flour, baking soda, and salt in a large bowl. Stir well.

Add the maple syrup, ghee, and eggs. Mix with a spoon until well incorporated with no remaining dry spots. Add the chocolate chips and stir again.

Divide the batter evenly among the 10 liners. Bake for 25-27 minutes, or until a toothpick inserted into the center of a muffin comes out clean. Serve warm or at room temperature.

Store leftovers, covered, at room temperature for 2 days, or longer in the refrigerator.

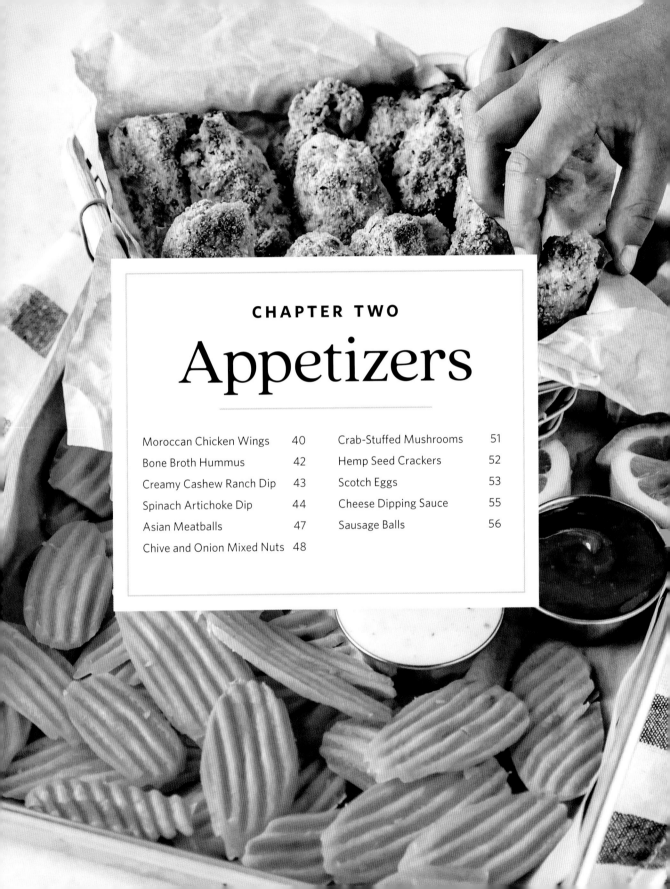

CHAPTER TWO
Appetizers

Moroccan Chicken Wings

YIELD: 4 TO 6 SERVINGS

The flavor of these wings is going to blow your dang mind. The Moroccan flavors I've infused into the wing sauce are just exquisite. You're going to want to serve these at any and all get-togethers. Or heck, do like I do and pair them with a big, juicy salad. Mm, mmm.

WINGS

2 ½ pounds (1.13 kg) chicken drumettes or wings

2 tablespoons (30 ml) avocado oil

1 teaspoon (6 g) kosher salt

½ teaspoon black pepper

SAUCE

¼ cup (60 ml) coconut aminos

¼ cup (60 ml) dry sherry

2 tablespoons (30 ml) avocado oil

2 tablespoons (30 ml) fresh lemon juice

2 tablespoons (30 ml) honey

4 cloves garlic, pressed

1 teaspoon (2 g) curry powder

½ teaspoon dried thyme

¼ teaspoon dried oregano

¼ teaspoon dried ginger

¼ teaspoon black pepper

1 ½ tablespoons (12 g) arrowroot flour

1 ½ tablespoons (22 ml) filtered water

⅓ cup (50 g) thinly sliced scallions, for garnish

Preheat the oven to 400°F (200°C) and adjust the oven rack to the middle position. Line a baking sheet with aluminum foil and top with a wire rack.

To make the wings, on a large cutting board, spread out the chicken in a single layer, skin side up. Using a paper towel, pat the skin as dry as you can.

Transfer the chicken to a large bowl. Add the oil, salt, and pepper. Toss to thoroughly coat.

Place the chicken on the wire rack. Make sure no chicken is touching. (If they are too close, they won't crisp.) Bake for 35 minutes. Turn the oven to a low broil and cook until crisp and golden, 5 minutes more.

Meanwhile, prepare the sauce. In a small saucepan, whisk together the coconut aminos, sherry, oil, lemon juice, honey, garlic, curry, thyme, oregano, ginger, and pepper. Cook over medium heat until it reaches a low boil. Turn down the heat to low and simmer for 15 to 20 minutes, stirring occasionally.

While the sauce is cooking, prepare an arrowroot slurry by combing the arrowroot flour with the water in a small bowl until smooth. During the last few minutes of sauce cook time, continue whisking while slowly pouring in enough slurry to reach your desired consistency.

When the wings are done, transfer them to a large bowl. Pour the sauce on top, mix, sprinkle with the scallions, and serve.

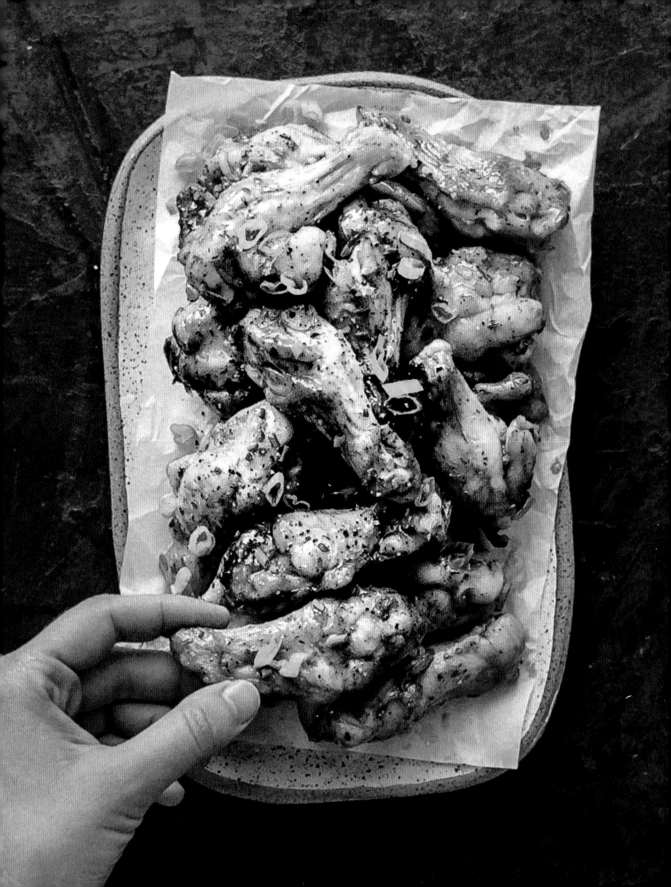

Bone Broth Hummus

YIELD: 1½ CUPS (340 G)

I am pretty sure that incorporating bone broth into my homemade dips and hummus is my favorite thing to do. It adds so much protein, flavor, and goodness that I can't resist. This hummus will become a staple in your refrigerator's snack drawer or one of the quickest and tastiest things you can bring to any potluck or get-together.

1 can (15 ounces [439 g]) chickpeas, drained, rinsed, and skins removed

½ cup (120 ml) beef or chicken bone broth

1 large lemon, juiced

¼ cup (56 g) creamy tahini, well stirred

2 ½ to 3 tablespoons (37 to 45 ml) olive oil or avocado oil

2 large cloves garlic

½ teaspoon ground cumin

1 teaspoon (6 g) kosher salt, plus more to taste

Black pepper, to taste

Combine the chickpeas in a saucepan with the bone broth. Bring to a simmer over medium-low heat and cook until the majority of the broth has been absorbed by the chickpeas, 3 to 5 minutes.

Transfer the mixture to a food processor or high-speed blender. Add the lemon juice, tahini, oil, garlic, cumin, and salt.

Process until smooth and creamy throughout, adding a tiny bit of oil as needed to smooth out completely.

Taste for additional salt and pepper, if you'd like.

Store in the refrigerator in an airtight container for up to 1 week.

Creamy Cashew Ranch Dip

YIELD: ABOUT 1 CUP (220 ML)

If you're looking for a tasty dip that will pair well with both cut veggies and chips, then look no further. Ranch dip is always a crowd favorite, and I'm always sure to bring it to a potluck or dinner party. This dip is satisfying without being too heavy.

1½ cups (225 g) raw cashews

⅓ cup (80 ml) chicken bone broth

⅓ cup (80 ml) filtered water

2 tablespoons (30 ml) fresh lemon juice

1 tablespoon (15 ml) coconut oil

1 tablespoon (8.5 g) nutritional yeast

1¼ teaspoons (3.8 g) garlic powder

½ teaspoon dried dill

Kosher salt, to taste

Black pepper, to taste

Place the cashews in a bowl and cover with boiling water. Set aside for 1½ hours. Drain and rinse well with cold water. Let drain thoroughly.

Transfer the cashews to the pitcher of a high-speed blender and add the broth, water, lemon juice, oil, nutritional yeast, garlic powder, dill, and a pinch of salt and pepper. Blend on high speed until it looks smooth and creamy. Depending on what type of blender you have, you may need to scrape down the sides a few times. Taste for salt and pepper.

Store in an airtight container in the refrigerator for up to 1 week.

Spinach Artichoke Dip

YIELD: 6 SERVINGS

This easy spinach artichoke dip is made with raw cashews, fresh spinach, coconut cream, and plenty of love. It's kid approved, and it pairs wonderfully with cut-up veggies, gluten-free bread, or other snacks. It's the perfect dip to have at a get-together, as it keeps well outside of the refrigerator, too!

1½ cups (225 g) raw cashews

¾ cup (180 ml) vegetable broth

¾ cup (180 ml) coconut cream (see Note)

¼ cup (15 g) nutritional yeast

1 lemon, juiced

1 teaspoon (6 g) kosher salt

1½ tablespoons (22 ml) avocado oil or coconut oil

1 shallot, sliced

8 cloves garlic, minced

2 cans (14 ounces [394 g]) artichoke hearts in water, drained

4 cups (141 g) loosely packed fresh spinach

Add the cashews to a bowl and cover with boiling water. Let sit, uncovered, for 1½ hours. Rinse and drain thoroughly.

Preheat the oven to 425°F (220°C) and adjust the oven rack to the middle position.

Transfer the cashews to a high-speed blender or food processor. Add the broth, coconut cream, nutritional yeast, lemon juice, and salt. Blend on high speed until smooth and creamy throughout, 1 to 2 minutes. You may need to scrape down the sides a few times or use a tamper.

In a medium skillet over medium-low heat, warm the oil. Once it is hot (about 1 minute), add the shallot and garlic. Sauté until fragrant and soft, stirring frequently, 2 to 3 minutes. Transfer the mixture to the blender.

Add the artichokes to the blender, along with the spinach. Pulse a few times or blend just until broken down a little bit. You want the mixture to be chunky, not smooth.

Transfer to a 2-quart (2 L) baking dish. Bake until the edges begin to turn golden brown, 22 to 26 minutes. You can turn the broiler on low at the end for a few minutes to speed up this process, too. Serve warm.

Note

Coconut cream is the cream that has separated and risen to the top of a can of full-fat coconut milk that has been refrigerated overnight. Alternatively, use cans of coconut cream, available in the ethnic foods section at the grocery store. Make sure it has at least 10 to 12 grams of fat for a super creamy and luscious dip.

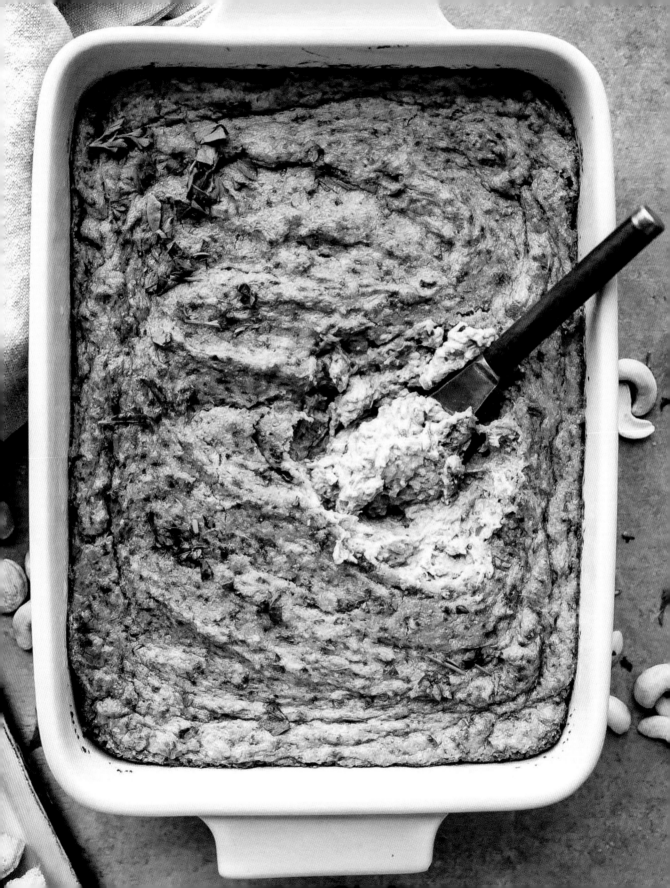

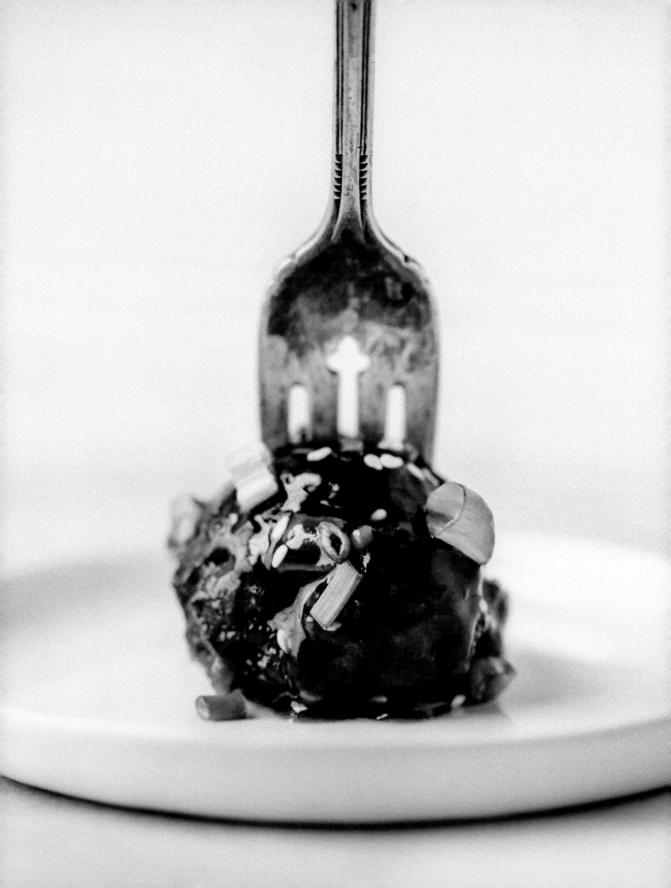

Asian Meatballs

YIELD: 18 TO 20 MEATBALLS

Who needs takeout when you can make these delicious meatballs with a sticky Asian sauce? It might take a little bit longer to make than it would to call in an order, but you'll have the satisfaction of knowing that there are no unhealthy ingredients here! Serve them with cauliflower rice and green beans to get the full takeout effect.

MEATBALLS

2 pounds (910 g) 90/10 ground beef

½ cup (48 g) almond flour

⅓ cup (53 g) chopped onion

1 large egg

1 tablespoon (15 ml) coconut aminos

½ teaspoon ground ginger

½ teaspoon ground garlic

½ teaspoon sea salt

2 large scallions, chopped, for garnish

Sesame seeds, for garnish

ASIAN STICKY SAUCE

1 cup (240 ml) coconut aminos

½ cup (120 ml) rice vinegar

1 ½ teaspoons sesame oil

1 clove garlic, minced

½ teaspoon ground ginger

1 tablespoon (6 g) arrowroot powder, dissolved in 1½ tablespoons (23 ml) water (see Note for keto)

Meatballs

Preheat the oven to 400°F (200°C or gas mark 6) and coat a baking sheet with olive oil or cooking spray.

Add the ground beef, almond flour, onion, egg, coconut aminos, ginger, garlic, salt, and pepper to a large bowl. Mix together with your hands until well combined. (Add a little more almond flour if the mixture is still too wet.)

Form the meatball mixture into golf ball–size balls; you should have 18 to 20. Place them on the prepared baking sheet.

Bake until the meatballs are browned and reach an internal temperature of 160°F (71°C), 20 to 25 minutes.

Asian Sticky Sauce

Place the coconut aminos, vinegar, sesame oil, garlic, and ginger in a small saucepan and set over medium-high heat.

Once the mixture is hot, add the dissolved arrowroot mixture. Reduce the heat to low and stir frequently. As the sauce heats, it will begin to thicken. This may take a few minutes.

Spoon the meatballs along with the sauce onto a plate. Serve sprinkled with the scallions and sesame seeds.

Note

You can substitute tapioca flour for arrowroot. If you're keto, use ¼ teaspoon xanthan gum or 1½ tablespoons (14 g) gelatin.

Chive and Onion Mixed Nuts

YIELD: 3½ CUPS (508 G)

These mixed nuts are the perfect snack or salad-topping option. They taste identical to a sour cream and onion potato chip—but without all the bad stuff.

3½ cups (508 g) unsalted mixed nuts (pecans, cashews, pistachios, almonds, and hazelnuts)

1½ tablespoons (23 ml) olive oil

1 tablespoon (2 g) dried chives

2 teaspoons onion powder

1 teaspoon garlic powder

1 teaspoon sea salt

Preheat the oven to 350°F (180°C or gas mark 4). Line a baking sheet with parchment paper.

In a large mixing bowl, combine the nuts with the olive oil, chives, onion powder, garlic powder, and salt. Mix together until the nuts are evenly coated.

Spread the nuts on the prepared baking sheet.

Bake until golden brown, about 10 to 13 minutes. Remove from the oven and allow the nuts to cool before serving. If desired, sprinkle a pinch of salt over all the nuts right when they come out of the oven.

Store in an airtight container for up to 2 weeks.

Note

Keep an eye on the nuts as they bake to make sure they don't burn. All ovens are different, so adjust the bake time as needed.

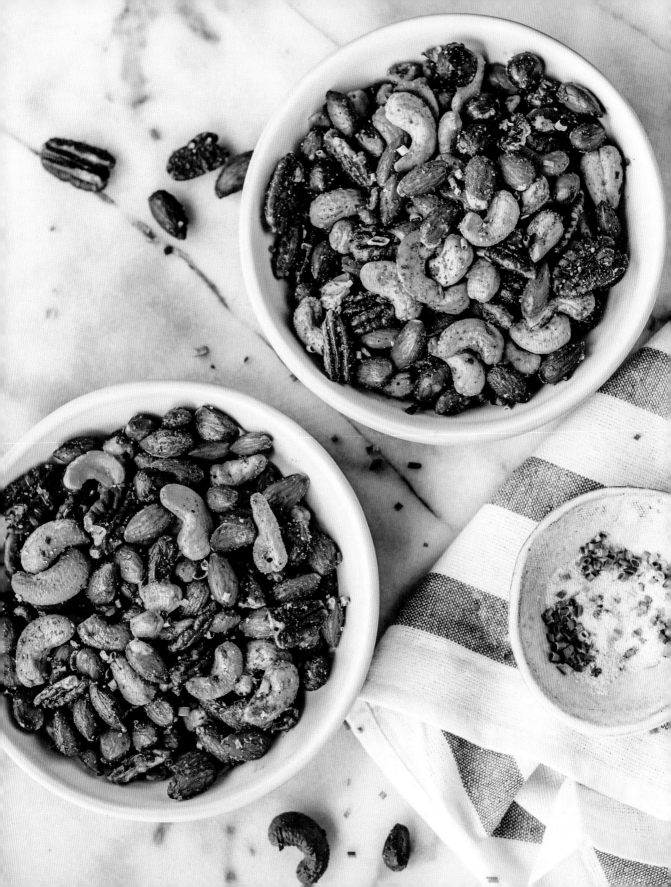

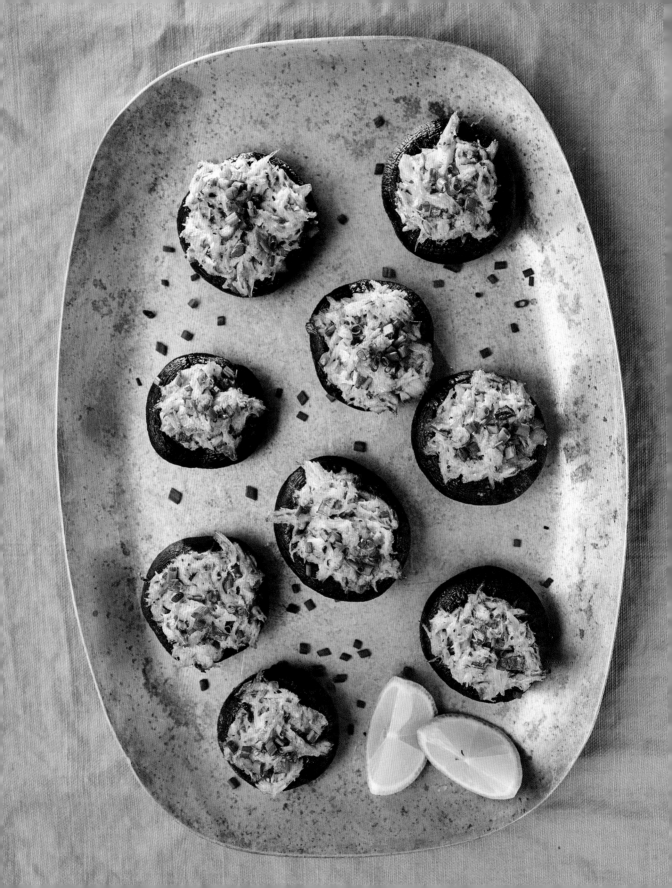

Crab-Stuffed Mushrooms

YIELD: 12 SERVINGS

The ultimate appetizer! These tender mushrooms are stuffed with a tasty crab-meat filling. They are easy and elegant.

Two 14-ounce (392 g) containers stuffing mushrooms (about 24 mushrooms)

1 tablespoon (15 ml) avocado oil

¼ cup (24 g) chopped green onion

¼ teaspoon salt

⅛ teaspoon pepper

Two 6-ounce (170 g) cans crabmeat, drained

¼ cup (60 ml) paleo mayonnaise

1 tablespoon (15 ml) lemon juice

½ teaspoon garlic powder

Preheat the oven to 350°F (180°C or gas mark 4).

Remove the stems from mushrooms and place them on a cutting board. Clean the mushrooms with a damp cloth or paper towel. Place them in a 13 by 9-inch (33 by 23 cm) pan.

Chop the mushroom stems and place them in a large skillet with the avocado oil, green onion, salt, and pepper. Cook for 5 minutes over medium heat.

While the mushroom mixture is cooking, place the crab in a medium-size bowl. Add the cooked mushroom mixture, mayo, lemon juice, and garlic powder and stir gently to combine but not break up the crabmeat. Scoop the mixture into the stuffing mushrooms.

Bake for 20–23 minutes, or until the mushrooms are tender. Serve immediately.

Hemp Seed Crackers

Making homemade crackers is easier than you think. These come out crunchy and are very hearty thanks to the seeds.

1 cup (160 g) shelled hemp seeds

1 cup (149 g) raw sun-flower seeds

1 large egg

1 tablespoon (15 ml) garlic-infused olive oil

2 teaspoons (5 g) Italian seasoning

¼ teaspoon salt

Preheat the oven to 300°F (150°C or gas mark 2). Line a baking sheet with parchment paper.

Combine the hemp seeds, sunflower seeds, egg, olive oil, Italian seasoning, and salt in a large bowl. Mix well.

Transfer the mixture to the prepared baking sheet and use your hands to press it into a 13 by 9-inch (33 by 23 cm) rectangle.

Bake for 20 minutes. Cut the crackers into 1-inch (3 cm) squares, separating them slightly, and bake for 10 more minutes.

Store leftovers, covered, at room temperature for up to 10 days.

Scotch Eggs

YIELD: 6 EGGS

This recipe makes perfectly cooked hard-boiled eggs wrapped in sausage. They are good warm or cold and are great for on the go!

6 hard-boiled eggs

1 pound (454 g) breakfast sausage, homemade or sugar-free store-bought

Preheat the oven to 350°F (180°C or gas mark 4). Line a baking sheet with parchment paper.

Peel the eggs and pat dry with a paper towel. Divide the sausage mixture into 6 equal portions, about ¼ cup (75 g) each. Roll a portion into a ball with your hands and then press it flat. Place an egg in the center of the sausage and form the meat around it. Squeeze the meat so it is packed on tightly. Place on the prepared baking sheet.

Repeat with the remaining eggs and sausage. Bake for 20–23 minutes, or until the meat is golden brown. Serve warm.

Store leftovers, covered, in the refrigerator for up to 6 days.

Note

I like to cook the eggs in the pressure cooker. Place them in the bottom with 1 cup (240 ml) of water and cook on high for 4 minutes. Do a quick release and place the eggs in a bowl of cold water for 3 minutes. Then they are ready to peel and be used.

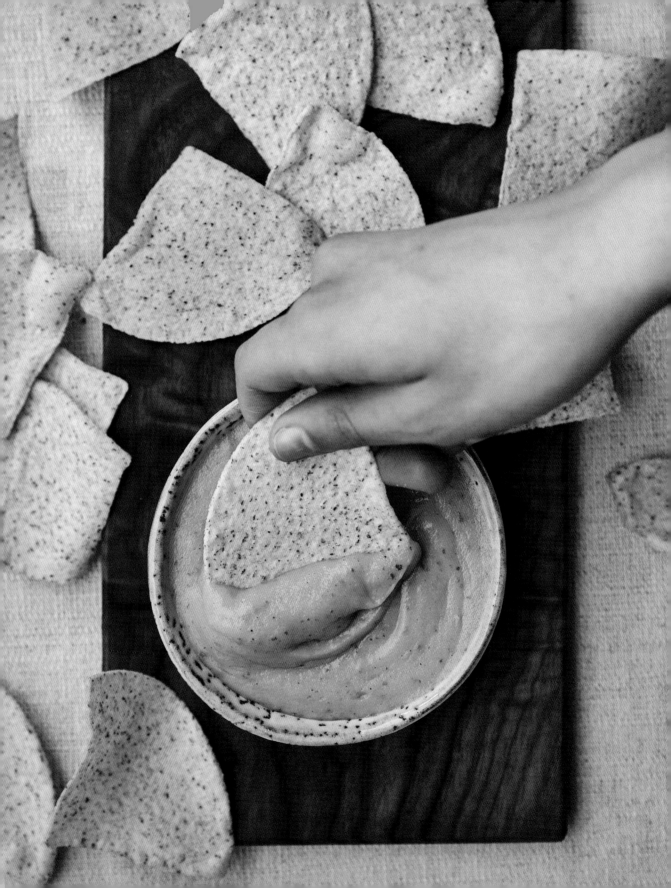

Cheese Dipping Sauce

YIELD: 3 CUPS (710 ML)

This dip is so smooth, it has the same consistency as melted cheese sauce. Grab some veggies, grain-free tortilla chips, or crackers and dig in!

1½ cups (192 g) chopped carrots (about 2 medium carrots)

2 cups (266 g) chopped potatoes (about 3 small russet potatoes)

1 teaspoon salt, divided

1 tablespoon (15 ml) garlic-infused olive oil

2 tablespoons (30 ml) lemon juice

2 tablespoons (30 g) ghee

¼ teaspoon ground black pepper

Place the carrots, potatoes, and ½ teaspoon of the salt in a large stockpot. Cover with water, cover the pot, and bring to a boil over high heat. Reduce the heat to medium and cook for about 15 minutes, or until the carrots and potatoes are tender.

Drain and transfer the vegetables to a high-powdered blender.

Add the olive oil, lemon juice, ghee, pepper, and remaining ½ teaspoon salt. Blend on high speed until smooth.

Serve as a dip with crackers, veggies, or chips. Or store leftovers, covered, in the refrigerator for up to a week. It will thicken as it cools; rewarm it if you want it thinner.

Sausage Balls

YIELD: 21 BALLS

This classic appetizer is made over to be gluten and dairy free. The baking soda in the sausage balls gives them a bubbly outside that is slightly crispy. Use any sausage you like for the spice level you desire.

1 pound (454 g) breakfast sausage, homemade or sugar-free store bought

1 cup (112 g) almond flour

1 teaspoon baking soda

Preheat the oven to 400°F (200°C or gas mark 6). Line a baking sheet with parchment paper.

Combine the sausage, almond flour, and baking soda in a large bowl. With your hands, scoop with a spoon into 1-inch (3 cm) balls, making about 21.

Arrange the balls on the prepared baking sheet and bake for 18–20 minutes, or until browned and crispy. Serve immediately.

Store leftovers, covered, in the refrigerator for up to 6 days.

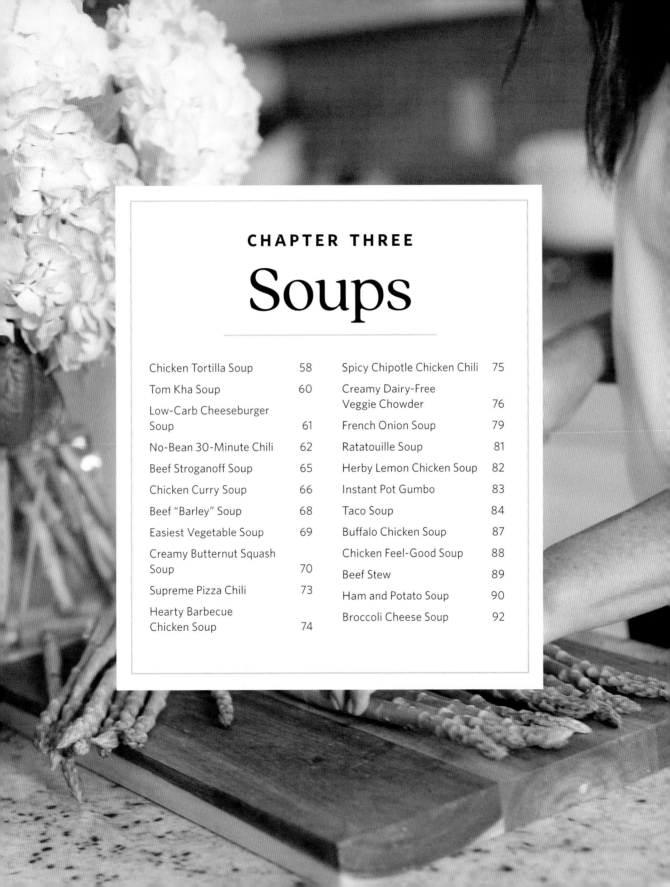

CHAPTER THREE
Soups

Chicken Tortilla Soup

YIELD: 6 SERVINGS

This warm and comforting soup is going to be your new go-to, especially after you see how simple it is to make. (Save time by using a rotisserie chicken!) The homemade tortilla strips are going to change your life, and I can almost assure you there won't be leftovers (for long, at least). If you already know you have no problem with black beans, you can absolutely throw in a can of those. Oh, and the creamy coconut milk mixed in really takes this soup to the next level, too.

TORTILLA STRIPS

¼ cup (60 ml) avocado oil

6 small corn tortillas, cut into ¼-inch (6 mm) strips

1 teaspoon (6 g) kosher salt

SOUP

2 tablespoons (30 ml) avocado oil

1 yellow onion, diced

1 jalapeño, minced (remove seeds for less heat)

6 cloves garlic, minced

1 quart (1 L) chicken broth or chicken bone broth (see Notes)

2 cans (14.5 ounces [435 ml]) diced tomatoes (see Notes)

3 cups (375 g) shredded cooked chicken

2 cups (250 g) corn kernels (see Notes)

½ lime, juiced

1 tablespoon (15 g) chili powder

1 to 2 teaspoons (6 to 12 g) kosher salt

1½ teaspoons (3.75 g) ground cumin

1½ teaspoons (7.5 g) smoked paprika

1 teaspoon (2 g) black pepper

⅔ cup (160 ml) full-fat canned coconut milk

Handful fresh cilantro, finely chopped

Diced avocado, for topping

To make the tortilla strips, place a large skillet over medium heat and warm the oil for 2 to 3 minutes, or until tiny bubbles start to form. Add the tortilla strips, taking care not to overcrowd them. Fry until crisp throughout, about 3 minutes, and transfer to a paper towel–lined plate. Sprinkle with the salt.

To make the soup, place a large Dutch oven or stockpot over medium-high heat and warm the oil for 2 minutes. Add the onion and jalapeño and sauté until they begin to soften, about 5 minutes. Add the garlic and sauté for another minute, stirring frequently.

Add the broth, tomatoes, chicken, corn, lime juice, chili powder, 1 teaspoon (5 g) salt, cumin, paprika, and pepper. Bring to a low boil and allow it to boil gently for 5 minutes, stirring occasionally. Add the coconut milk and return to a low boil. Cook for an additional 3 to 5 minutes, stirring occasionally. Add the cilantro and boil for 1 minute more.

Taste and add more salt, if needed.

Ladle the soup into bowls and top with the tortilla strips, avocado, and more cilantro, if desired.

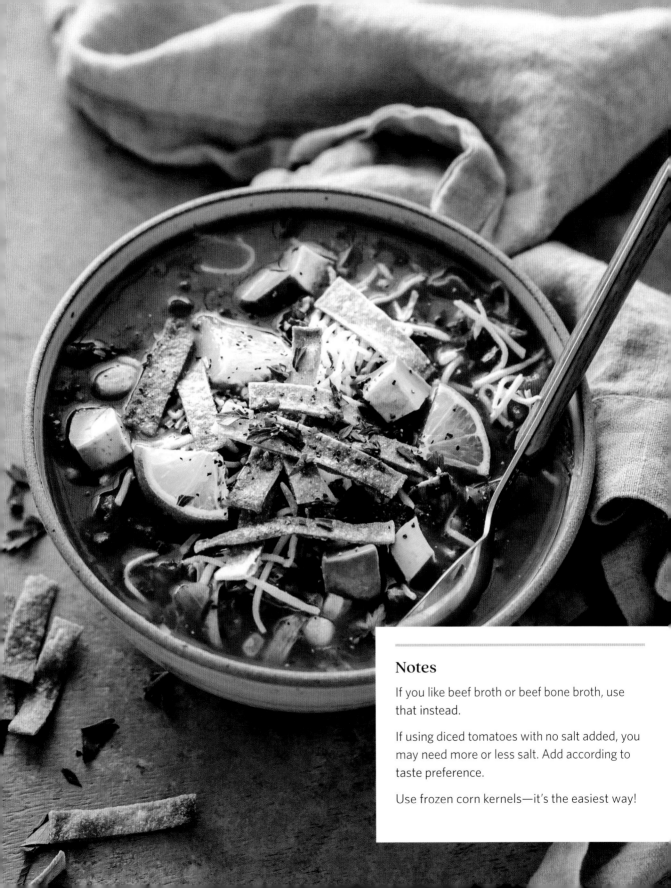

Notes

If you like beef broth or beef bone broth, use that instead.

If using diced tomatoes with no salt added, you may need more or less salt. Add according to taste preference.

Use frozen corn kernels—it's the easiest way!

Tom Kha Soup

YIELD: 6 TO 8 SERVINGS

Tom kha is a flavorful Thai soup that is spicy and sour and made with a coconut milk base. It takes very little time to prep, and you can dump everything into one pot, which is a huge bonus! You're going to love this tangy, salty soup full of delectable shrimp. Don't skimp on those Thai chiles, as they infuse a ton of flavor and fabulous heat! Serve it by itself or pour over rice or cauliflower rice.

3 cans (13.5 ounces [395 ml]) full-fat coconut milk

1 quart (1 L) chicken bone broth or low-sodium chicken broth (see Notes)

6 to 8 Thai chiles, depending on heat preferences (see Notes)

1½ -inch (3.75 cm) knob fresh ginger, peeled and minced

8 ounces (230 g) cremini or baby bella mushrooms, thinly sliced

2 pounds (900 g) large shrimp, peeled and deveined

2 limes, juiced

2½ tablespoons (37 ml) fish sauce

2½ tablespoons (37 ml) coconut aminos

Kosher salt, to taste

Black pepper, to taste

Coarsely chopped fresh cilantro, for serving

Lime wedges, for serving

In a large pot or Dutch oven, bring the coconut milk and broth to a boil over medium-high heat. Lower the heat to medium and add the Thai chiles and ginger. Simmer for 10 minutes.

Add the mushrooms and simmer, stirring occasionally, for 5 minutes.

Add the shrimp, lime juice, fish sauce, and coconut aminos. Simmer until the shrimp are cooked through, about 5 minutes.

Taste and add more Thai chiles if it is not spicy enough for you. Continue simmering for another 10 minutes.

Check for seasoning, adding salt and black pepper if necessary. Add even more Thai chiles, if you'd like.

Top off the soup with chopped cilantro and serve with fresh lime wedges.

Notes

I recommend using bone broth if you have access to it. However, chicken broth is a fine substitute.

Taste the soup regularly and add more Thai chiles if the soup isn't spicy enough for you. I end up using a large handful!

Low-Carb Cheeseburger Soup

YIELD: 8 SERVINGS

If I told you you could have all the fabulous flavors of a cheeseburger in a nutritious and dairy-free soup, would you believe me? Well, this creamy cheeseburger soup is made rich with cashews, bacon, and bone broth. It also has plenty of broccoli because we all need our vegetables, don't we? You're going to love this so much, you won't even miss the cheese (or the bun!).

1½ cups (225 g) raw cashews

6 strips bacon, diced

2 pounds (900 g) grass-fed 90 / 10 ground beef

2½ cups (595 ml) beef bone broth

1 can (13.5 ounces [395 ml]) full-fat coconut milk

1 can (6 ounces [180 g]) tomato paste

2 teaspoons (12 g) kosher salt

1½ pounds (680 g) broccoli florets

Black pepper, to taste

Sliced avocado, for garnish

Fresh parsley, for garnish

Add the cashews to a bowl and cover with boiling water. Let sit, uncovered, for 1½ hours. Drain the soaked cashews and rinse well with cold water. Set aside.

In a large pot, cook the bacon pieces over medium heat until crispy, 3 to 4 minutes. Increase the heat to medium-high and add the ground beef. Cook, stirring often to break the beef apart into even pieces, until it is brown throughout, 8 to 10 minutes.

Meanwhile, in the pitcher of a high-speed blender, add the broth, coconut milk, tomato paste, drained cashews, and salt. Blend on high speed until smooth and creamy throughout.

Transfer the cashew mixture to the pot and stir well. Bring to a boil over medium-high heat, stirring occasionally.

Reduce the heat to a simmer, add the broccoli florets, and cook until the broccoli is fork-tender, another 10 to 15 minutes. Taste for seasoning (salt and pepper) and remove from the heat. Serve topped with avocado and parsley—or your preferred cheeseburger toppings!

No-Bean 30-Minute Chili

YIELD: 6 TO 8 SERVINGS

This yummy chili is thick. It's hearty. It's dark. It doesn't have beans, but you're not going to notice. It's a chili you are going to want to make on a regular basis.

PALEO SIMPLE

2 pounds (900 g) lean ground beef or turkey

1 green bell pepper, finely chopped

1 large yellow onion, finely chopped

2 cans (14.5 ounces, or 410 g, each) diced tomatoes

2 cups (475 ml) beef stock

1 can (6 ounces, or 170 g) tomato paste

¼ cup (40 g) minced garlic

1½ tablespoons (12 g) chili powder

1½ teaspoons paprika

1½ teaspoons onion powder

1½ teaspoons salt

1 teaspoon garlic powder

1 teaspoon ground cumin

1 teaspoon black pepper

Sliced scallions, diced onion, chopped avocado, or chopped cilantro, for garnish

Add the ground beef or turkey to a soup pot over medium-high heat. Use a spatula to crumble.

Add the bell pepper and onion. Cook, stirring occasionally, until the beef is browned and the veggies are softened, about 5 minutes.

Add the tomatoes, stock, tomato paste, garlic, chili powder, paprika, onion powder, salt, garlic powder, cumin, and black pepper. Stir. Reduce the heat to medium, cover, and simmer until the flavors marry, about 20 minutes.

Taste and add extra salt or black pepper, if you like. Serve with desired toppings.

Note

If your meat isn't very lean, you'll want to drain the grease after browning it. I use a 93% lean beef, so I don't drain mine.

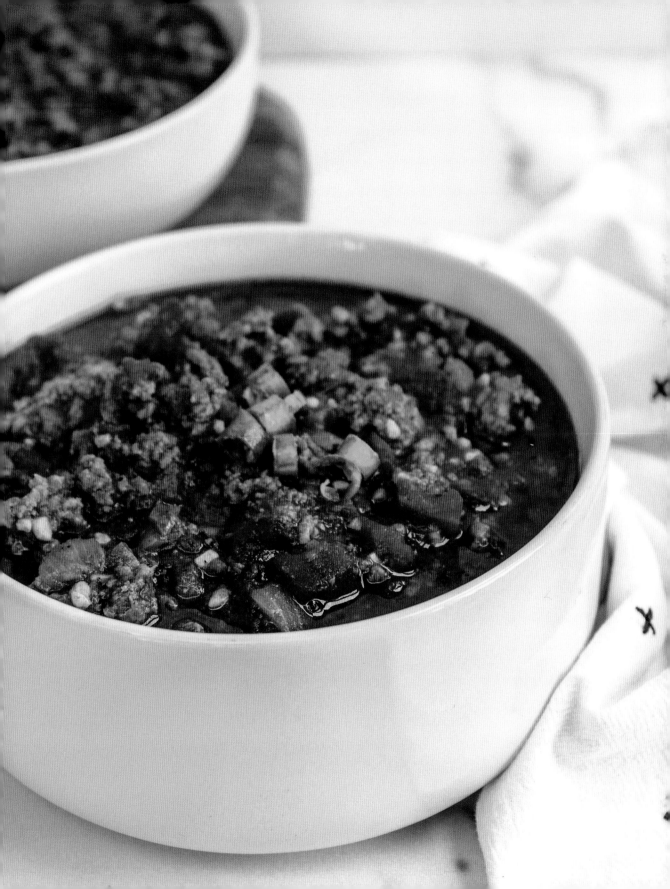

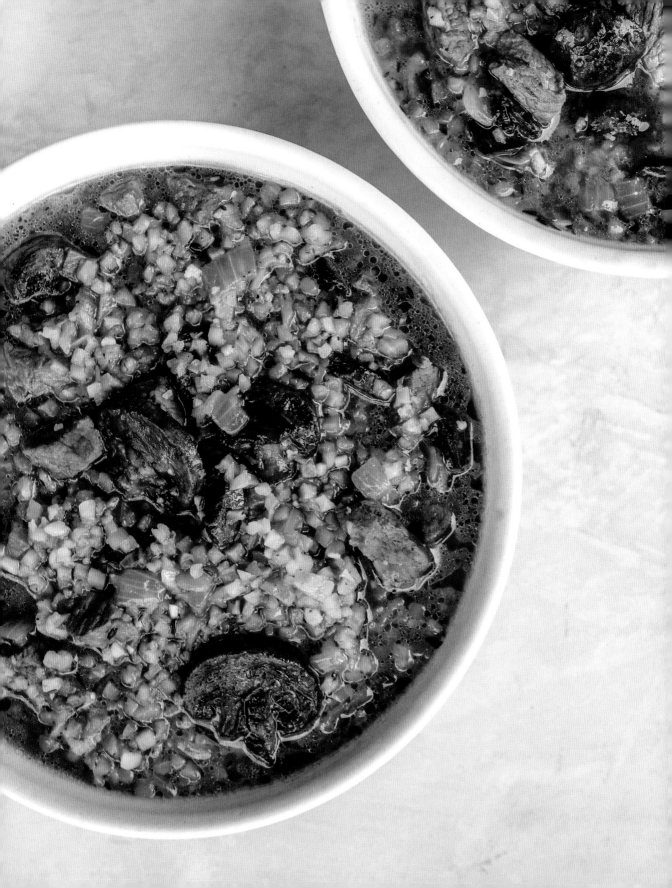

Beef Stroganoff Soup

YIELD: 6 TO 8 SERVINGS

This soup has all the flavor of a classic beef stroganoff, but it's oh so much lighter! It's rich, creamy, and tastes like it has been simmering for ages. I can't wait for you to try it!

1 tablespoon (15 ml) extra-virgin olive oil or ghee (For dairy-free dishes, use extra-virgin olive oil.)

1 pound (455 g) sirloin steak, sliced into small pieces

8 ounces (225 g) sliced mushrooms

½ white or yellow onion, diced into ½-inch (1 cm) pieces

2 teaspoons minced garlic

32 ounces (946 ml) beef stock

⅔ cup (160 ml) unsweetened, full-fat coconut milk, stirred

1 teaspoon balsamic vinegar

¾ teaspoon salt

½ teaspoon black pepper

½ teaspoon dried thyme

2 cups (8 ounces, or 225 g) cauliflower rice

Add the oil or ghee to your soup pot over medium-high heat. Once hot, add the steak, mushrooms, onion, and garlic. Sauté until the onion becomes tender and the steak is beautifully browned, about 5 minutes.

Add the stock, coconut milk, vinegar, salt, black pepper, and thyme. Cover, reduce the heat to medium, and simmer for 10 minutes.

Stir in the cauliflower rice. Cover and continue to simmer until the cauliflower is tender, another 10 minutes.

Note

The coconut milk helps create a creaminess in this soup that's reminiscent of traditional beef stroganoff. You will not taste any coconut in this dish since we're not using much, and I've paired it with plenty of other bold flavors that overpower it.

SOUPS

Chicken Curry Soup

YIELD: 6 TO 8 SERVINGS

Craving all the flavor of curry but want it fast? This soup features a creamy curry broth, chicken, bell peppers, and sweet potato. It's a simple dish that packs tons of flavor.

2 tablespoons (28 ml) extra-virgin olive oil or avocado oil

2 red bell peppers, diced into ½-inch (1 cm) pieces

1 white or yellow onion, diced into ½-inch (1 cm) pieces

1 teaspoon minced garlic

1½ pounds (680 g) boneless, skinless chicken breasts, cut into 1-inch (2.5 cm) pieces

2 cups (266 g) diced sweet potatoes, 1-inch (2.5 cm) cubes

32 ounces (946 ml) chicken stock

1 can (14.5 ounces, or 410 g) diced tomatoes

¼ cup (64 g) tomato paste

1 tablespoon (6 g) curry powder

1 teaspoon ground ginger

1 teaspoon salt

½ teaspoon cayenne pepper

¼ teaspoon ground cumin

¼ teaspoon coriander

1 can (13.5 ounces, or 380 g) unsweetened full-fat coconut milk

Fresh cilantro, chopped

Add the oil to your soup pot over medium-high heat. Once hot, add the bell peppers and onion. Sauté until the onion is tender, 3 to 5 minutes. Add the garlic and sauté for another minute so the garlic is golden in color.

Add the chicken, sweet potatoes, stock, tomatoes, tomato paste, curry powder, ginger, salt, cayenne pepper, cumin, and coriander. Bring to a boil over high heat. Cover and reduce the heat to medium. Simmer until the chicken is cooked through and the sweet potato is tender, 15 to 20 minutes.

Remove from the heat and stir in the coconut milk. Top with fresh chopped cilantro when you're ready to serve!

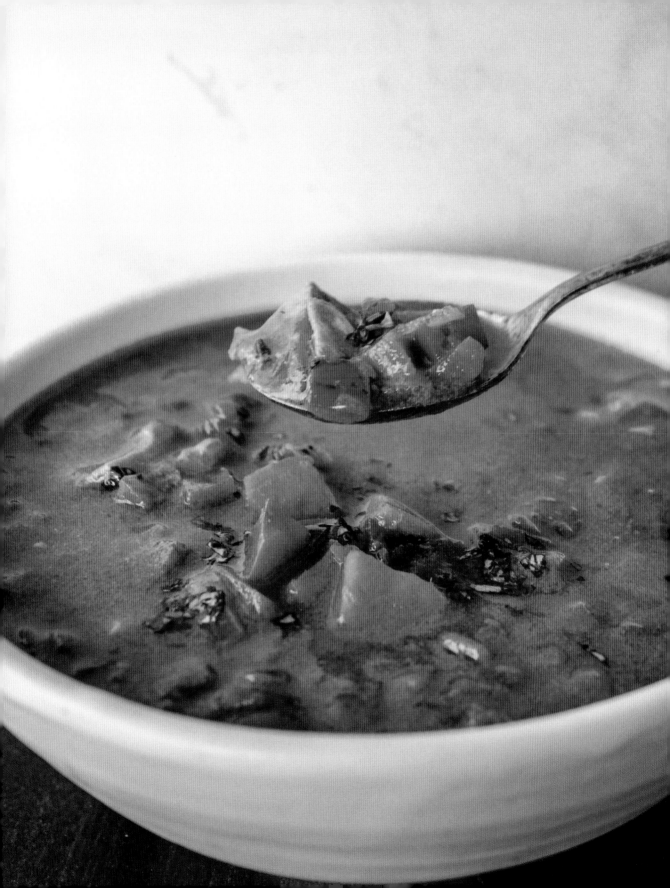

Beef "Barley" Soup

Is there barley in here? No, it's cauliflower rice! It's a perfect swap because it really looks so much like barley and absorbs whatever flavors you cook it with. Steak, veggies, and a tasty broth make this soup a complete meal.

1½ tablespoons (25 ml) extra-virgin olive oil or ghee (For dairy-free dishes, use extra-virgin olive oil.)

1 to 1½ pounds (455 to 680 g) sirloin steak, sliced into small pieces

½ white or yellow onion, diced into ½-inch (1 cm) pieces

1 cup (120 g) diced celery, ½-inch (1 cm) dice

1 cup (70 g) sliced mushrooms

1 cup (122 g) peeled, sliced carrots, ¼-inch (6 mm)-thick slices

1 tablespoon (10 g) minced garlic

32 ounces (946 ml) beef stock

2 tablespoons (32 g) tomato paste

2 tablespoons (28 ml) balsamic vinegar

2 teaspoons salt

1½ teaspoons black pepper

1 teaspoon dried thyme

1 teaspoon dried rosemary

1 teaspoon dried oregano

3 cups (12 ounces, or 340 g) fresh or frozen cauliflower rice

Add the oil or ghee and steak to your soup pot over medium-high heat. Brown all sides of the steak pieces, 3 to 4 minutes. Remove from the pot and set aside.

Add the onion, celery, mushrooms, carrots, and garlic to the pot. You should have enough fat from the beef already remaining, but add another 1½ teaspoons oil if not. Sauté until the onion becomes tender and fragrant, about 4 minutes.

Add the steak back to the pot along with the stock, tomato paste, vinegar, salt, black pepper, thyme, rosemary, and oregano. Reduce the heat to medium, cover, and simmer for 10 minutes.

Stir in the cauliflower rice. Cover and simmer until the cauliflower is soft, 8 to 10 minutes.

Easiest Vegetable Soup

YIELD: 6 TO 8 SERVINGS

A truly delicious homemade vegetable soup doesn't need any meat at all. Mine is full of fresh veggies, including green beans, carrots, and sweet potatoes. They're swimming in a rich broth that will keep you coming back for more.

1 tablespoon (15 ml) extra-virgin olive oil or avocado oil

½ large white or yellow onion, diced into ½-inch (1 cm) pieces

1 teaspoon minced garlic

32 ounces (946 ml) chicken or vegetable stock (For vegan and vegetarian dishes, use vegetable stock.)

1 can (14.5 ounces, or 410 g) diced tomatoes

1 cup (100 g) chopped green beans

1 cup (122 g) peeled, sliced carrots, ¼-inch (6 mm)-thick slices

1 cup (133 g) diced sweet potatoes, ½-inch (1 cm) cubes

½ teaspoon salt

½ teaspoon black pepper

1 packed cup (about half a 5-ounce, or 140 g, package) baby spinach

¼ cup (15 g) chopped fresh parsley

Add the oil to your soup pot over medium to medium-high heat. Once the oil is hot, add the onion and sauté until softened, 3 to 4 minutes. Add the garlic and sauté for another minute so the garlic is golden in color.

Add the stock, tomatoes, green beans, carrots, sweet potatoes, salt, and black pepper. Bring to a boil over high heat. Cover, reduce the heat to medium, and simmer until the veggies are tender, 15 to 20 minutes.

Stir in the spinach and parsley. They will wilt right away. Taste and add extra salt or black pepper, if desired.

Creamy Butternut Squash Soup

YIELD: 6 SERVINGS

This butternut squash soup is velvety smooth and creamy—but without the cream! The squash tastes like it's been roasted, but to keep things simple, we sauté it with carrots, onion, and garlic. This easy step brings out all its scrumptious flavor in very little time. If fall were a soup, it would be this one!

4 tablespoons (60 ml) extra-virgin olive oil or avocado oil, divided

3 carrots, peeled and sliced, ¼-inch (6 mm)-thick slices

½ white or yellow onion, diced into ½-inch (1 cm) pieces

1 tablespoon (10 g) minced garlic

2 pounds (900 g) butternut squash, peeled and cut into 1-inch (2.5 cm) cubes (see Notes)

3 to 4 cups (700 to 946 ml) chicken or vegetable stock (see Notes) (For vegan and vegetarian dishes, use vegetable stock.)

¾ teaspoon salt

½ teaspoon ground cinnamon

½ teaspoon ground nutmeg

Canned unsweetened coconut milk, for garnish (optional)

Add 2 tablespoons (28 ml) of the oil to a large skillet over medium-high heat. Once hot, add the carrots and onion. Sauté until the carrots are tender, 6 to 8 minutes. Add the garlic and sauté for another minute so the garlic is golden in color. Transfer to a high-powered blender. Set aside.

Add the remaining 2 tablespoons (28 ml) oil to the skillet, along with the butternut squash, and return to medium-high heat. Cover and cook, stirring occasionally, until the squash is tender and has some beautiful browning, about 10 minutes. Transfer to the blender. Add the stock, salt, cinnamon, and nutmeg. Blend until smooth. (You may need to work in batches, depending on the size of your blender.)

Taste and add more salt, if desired. Pour or ladle into bowls and top with a drizzle of coconut milk, if desired, to make it look extra special.

Note

For a thick soup, use 3 cups (700 ml) stock. For a thinner soup, use 4 cups (946 ml).

Cut the butternut squash into cubes ¾ to 1 inch (2 to 2.5 cm) big. Some grocery stores carry prechopped squash in this very size. It's a huge time-saver!

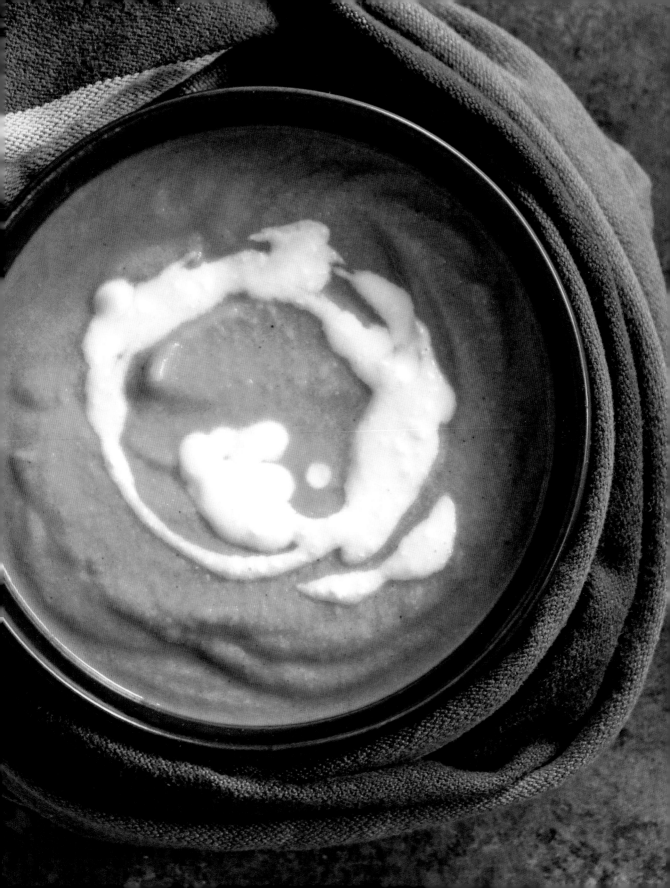

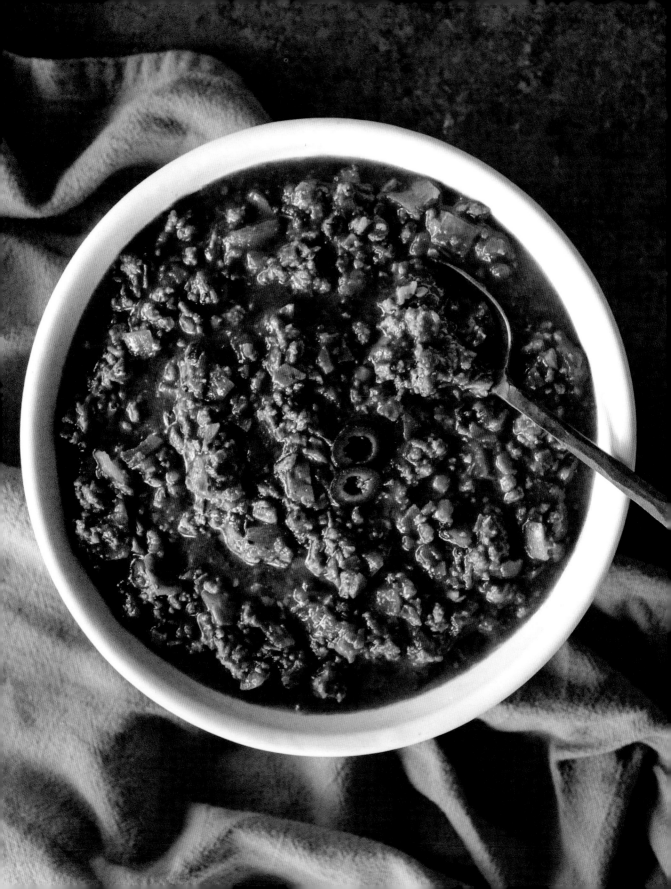

Supreme Pizza Chili

YIELD: 6 SERVINGS

Supreme pizza in a bowl? If it sounds strange, you're in for a surprise. Beef, onion, pepperoni, olives (yes, olives!), tomatoes, bell pepper, and mushrooms make this fun chili really taste like a supreme pizza!

1 pound (455 g) 93% lean ground beef

½ white or yellow onion, diced into ½-inch (1 cm) pieces

1 teaspoon minced garlic

3 cups (700 ml) beef stock

1 can (14.5 ounces, or 410 g) diced tomatoes

1 cup (138 g) finely diced pepperoni (see Note)

1 cup (70 g) sliced mushrooms

½ green bell pepper, diced into ½-inch (1 cm) pieces

3 tablespoons (48 g) tomato paste

2 tablespoons (12 g) Italian seasoning

1½ tablespoons (9 g) chopped black olives

1 teaspoon salt

½ teaspoon black pepper

Add your ground beef to a soup pot over medium-high heat. Use your spatula to crumble and add in the onion. Cook, stirring occasionally, until the beef is browned. Add the garlic and sauté for another minute so the garlic is golden in color. (If your beef isn't giving you enough fat to sauté the onion, add 1 tablespoon [15 ml] oil.)

Add the stock, tomatoes, pepperoni, mushrooms, bell pepper, tomato paste, Italian seasoning, olives, salt, and black pepper. Stir, cover, reduce the heat to medium, and simmer until the peppers are tender and the flavors have married, 15 to 20 minutes. Taste and add extra salt or black pepper if you like.

Note

Check the ingredients in your pepperoni! The one I prefer is actually made of turkey instead of pork and can be found in the natural foods section of higher-end grocery stores or in natural foods stores.

Hearty Barbecue Chicken Soup

YIELD: 6 SERVINGS

This thick soup has a flavor that is reminiscent of a lightly sweetened honey-barbecue sauce. It's a surprising twist on chicken soup! And, it's ready in about 20 minutes because we start with cooked shredded chicken (use leftover chicken or buy a rotisserie chicken!).

1 tablespoon (15 ml) extra-virgin olive oil or avocado oil

½ white or yellow onion, diced into ½-inch (1 cm) pieces

1 teaspoon minced garlic

2 cups (475 ml) chicken stock

2 cups (250 g) shredded cooked chicken

1 can (14.5 ounces, or 410 g) fire-roasted diced tomatoes

1 can (6 ounces, or 170 g) tomato paste

3 to 4 tablespoons (60 to 85 g) raw honey

1 teaspoon chili powder

½ teaspoon paprika

½ teaspoon salt

½ teaspoon black pepper

Add the oil to your soup pot over medium-high heat. Once hot, add the onion and sauté until tender with some browning, about 3 minutes. When the onion is almost done, stir in the garlic. Sauté for about 1 minute so that it has a bit of a golden color.

Add the stock, chicken, tomatoes, tomato paste, 3 tablespoons (60 g) honey, chili powder, paprika, salt, and black pepper. Stir, reduce the heat to medium, cover, and simmer until heated through, about 10 minutes.

Taste. Add more honey if you want it sweeter or salt and black pepper if you want to amp up the savory flavor a bit.

Spicy Chipotle Chicken Chili

YIELD: 6 TO 8 SERVINGS

This is not a mild chili. Oh no, this one has some spiciness that really sets it apart!

1½ tablespoons (25 ml) extra-virgin olive oil or avocado oil

2 red bell peppers, diced into ½-inch (1 cm) pieces

1 white or yellow onion, diced into ½-inch (1 cm) pieces

2 teaspoons minced garlic

2 cups (475 ml) chicken stock

1¾ to 2 pounds (795 to 900 g) boneless, skinless chicken breasts, cut into 1-inch (2.5 cm) pieces (see Note)

1 can (28 ounces, or 785 g) diced tomatoes

1 can (6 ounces, or 170 g) tomato paste

1½ tablespoons (11 g) chili powder

1½ teaspoons paprika

1 teaspoon chipotle chili powder

1 teaspoon salt

1 teaspoon black pepper

¾ teaspoon ground cumin

½ teaspoon onion powder

½ teaspoon garlic powder

Add the oil to your soup pot over medium-high heat. Add the bell peppers and onion. Sauté until tender with some browning, 3 to 5 minutes. Add the garlic and let everything sauté for about another minute until the garlic turns a golden color.

Add the stock, chicken, tomatoes, tomato paste, chili powder, paprika, chipotle powder, salt, black pepper, cumin, onion powder, and garlic powder. Bring to a boil over high heat. Cover, reduce the heat to medium-high or medium, and simmer until the chicken is cooked through, completely opaque and juices run clear, about 15 minutes.

Taste and add extra salt or black pepper if you like.

Note

If you have a bit more time, keep the chicken breasts whole and simmer until cooked through to a minimum internal temperature of 165°F (74°C), 20 to 25 minutes. Remove to a cutting board, use two forks to shred, and mix back into the chili. I like having shredded chicken in my chili, so I prefer to do it this way when time permits.

Creamy Dairy-Free Veggie Chowder

YIELD: 6 SERVINGS

This thick, smooth chowder gives you veggies, veggies, and more veggies. We blend cauliflower with all the best aromatics for a creamy soup base you will swear includes dairy (but doesn't). If you fantasize about vegetables, this is the soup you want!

4 tablespoons (60 ml) extra-virgin olive oil or avocado oil, divided

4 cups (16 ounces, or 455 g) cauliflower rice

½ white or yellow onion, coarsely chopped

1 tablespoon (10 g) minced garlic

2½ to 3 cups (570 to 700 ml) vegetable stock (see Note)

½ cup (120 ml) unsweetened full-fat coconut milk, stirred

1 teaspoon salt

5 carrots, peeled and sliced ¼-inch (6 mm) thick (about 1½ cups, or 183 g)

5 ribs celery, chopped (about 1½ cups, or 150 g)

1 medium zucchini, halved and cut into half-moons (about 1½ cups, or 180 g)

½ bunch asparagus, trimmed and cut into thirds or fourths (about 2 cups, or 268 g)

Add 2 tablespoons (28 ml) of the oil to a soup pot over medium-high heat. Once hot, add the cauliflower rice, onion, and garlic. Cover and cook, stirring occasionally, until the cauliflower and onion are tender, 6 to 8 minutes. Transfer to a high-powered blender along with the stock, coconut milk, and salt. If using an immersion blender, transfer to a mixing bowl. Blend until smooth. Set aside.

Add the remaining 2 tablespoons (28 ml) oil to the pot. When hot, add the carrots, celery, zucchini, and asparagus. (If your asparagus has especially thin stalks, add them in the last 3 minutes of your cooking time instead of here.) Cover and sauté over medium-high (or medium) heat, stirring occasionally, until the carrots are tender, 6 to 8 minutes.

Pour the creamy soup back into the pot with the veggies. Stir and simmer for 2 to 3 minutes so everything is warm. Taste and add extra salt, if desired.

Note

For a thick soup, use 2½ cups (570 ml) vegetable stock. If you'd prefer a thinner consistency, use 3 cups (700 ml).

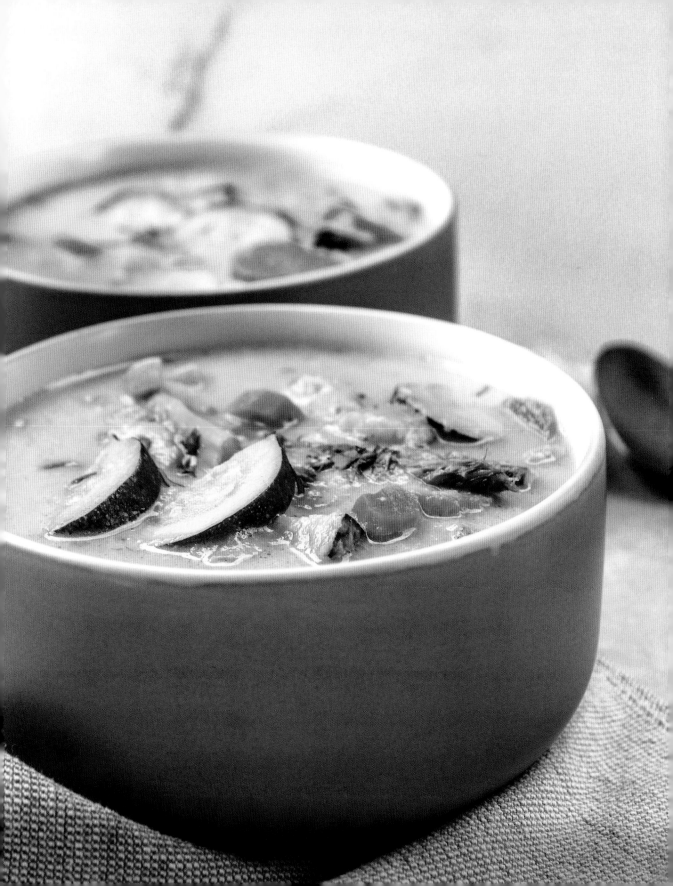

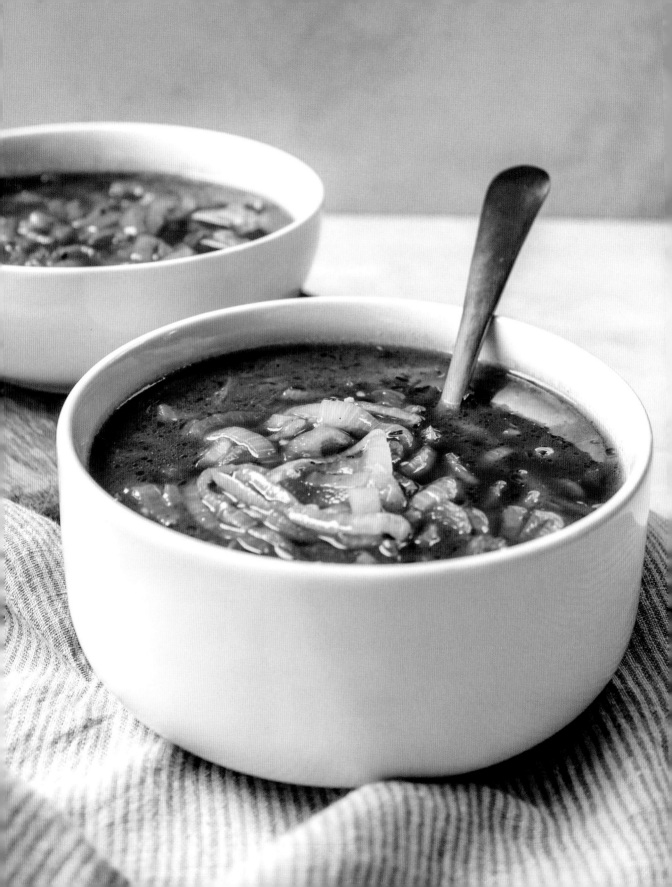

French Onion Soup

A rich French onion soup can take upwards of an hour to make. Allowing the onions and garlic to caramelize is really where all the magic happens. This is what creates that rich flavor we know and love! To keep the cook time short, I add a hit of flavor with balsamic vinegar; you won't believe it's done in 30 minutes. Enjoy this easy French onion soup as a meal or delicious side.

¼ cup (56 g) ghee or cooking fat of choice (For dairy-free dishes, do not use ghee.)

3 pounds (1.4 kg) yellow onions, sliced

2 tablespoons (20 g) minced garlic

6 cups (1.4 L) beef stock

3 to 4 tablespoons (45 to 60 ml) balsamic vinegar (see Note)

2 bay leaves

1 teaspoon chopped fresh thyme

1 teaspoon salt

1 teaspoon black pepper

¼ teaspoon onion powder

¼ teaspoon garlic powder

Add the ghee to your soup pot over medium-high heat. Once hot, add the onions and garlic. Sauté, stirring frequently, until the onion is wilted with some browning, about 10 minutes. You can cover for the last minute to speed up the process.

Add the stock, 3 tablespoons (45 ml) of vinegar, bay leaves, thyme, salt, black pepper, onion powder, and garlic powder. Cover, reduce the heat to medium, and simmer until the onions are tender and the flavors marry, 10 to 15 minutes.

Taste and add extra salt, black pepper, or vinegar if you like. Remove the bay leaves before serving.

Note

Balsamic vinegar is powerful, but it adds a sweetness I enjoy in place of wine in savory dishes. Start with 3 tablespoons (45 ml) and add another tablespoon (15 ml) after tasting, if desired.

SOUPS

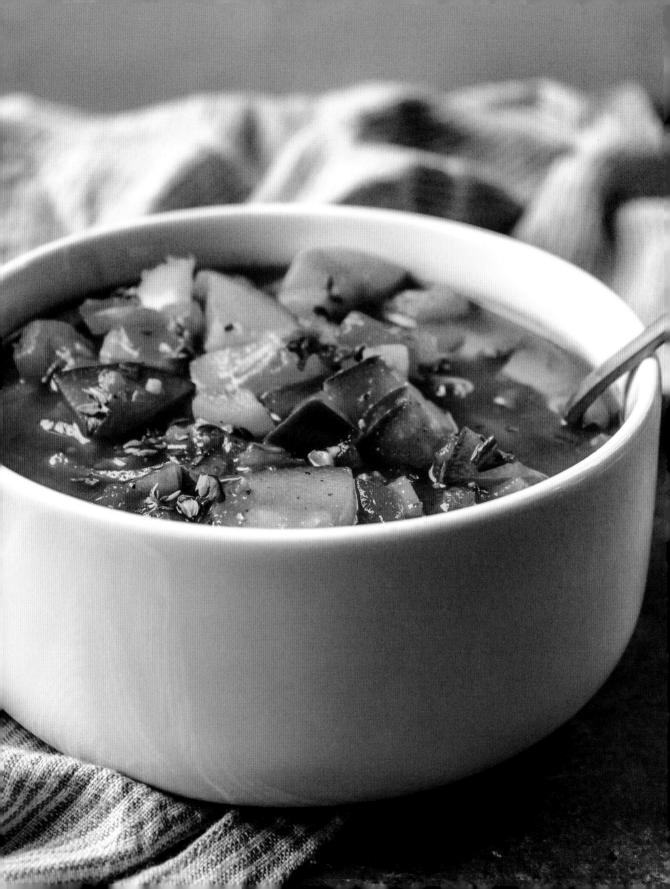

Ratatouille Soup

YIELD: 6 TO 8 SERVINGS

Ratatouille is a French dish of stewed or roasted vegetables that takes a lot of time to prepare. We're switching things up and enjoying it as a soup to keep it fast but still a celebration of beautifully prepared fresh produce. Dice all your vegetables into ½-inch (1 cm) pieces so you'll have a bit of everything in each spoonful.

3 tablespoons (45 ml) extra-virgin olive oil or avocado oil, divided

1 red bell pepper, diced

1 yellow bell pepper, diced

1 white or yellow onion, diced

1 tablespoon (1 g) minced garlic

1 cup (82 g) diced eggplant

1 cup (120 g) diced yellow squash

1 cup (120 g) diced zucchini

32 ounces (946 ml) vegetable stock

2 cups (360 g) diced tomatoes

2 tablespoons (32 g) tomato paste

1 teaspoon salt

½ teaspoon black pepper

¼ teaspoon crushed red pepper flakes (optional)

2 tablespoons (8 g) chopped fresh parsley

Add 2 tablespoons (28 ml) of the oil to your soup pot over medium-high heat. Add the bell peppers and onion. Sauté until tender with some browning, 3 to 5 minutes. Add the garlic and sauté for about another minute until the garlic turns a golden color.

Add the eggplant, squash, and zucchini along with the remaining 1 tablespoon (15 ml) oil. Stir and give these veggies a quick sauté, about 2 minutes, just to bring out their flavors a bit more. We're not cooking them through here.

Add the stock, tomatoes, tomato paste, salt, black pepper, and red pepper flakes (if using). Cover, reduce the heat to medium, and simmer until the vegetables are tender, 10 to 15 minutes.

Stir in the chopped fresh parsley. Taste and add extra salt or black pepper if you like.

Herby Lemon Chicken Soup

YIELD: 6 TO 8 SERVINGS

A lemony broth and fresh herbs will have you coming back for more of this chicken soup. It's delightful any time of year!

1½ tablespoons (25 ml) extra-virgin olive oil or avocado oil

½ white or yellow onion, diced into ½-inch (1 cm) pieces

1 cup (120 g) diced celery, ½-inch (1 cm) dice

1 tablespoon (10 g) minced garlic

32 ounces (946 ml) chicken stock

1½ pounds (680 g) boneless, skinless chicken breasts or thighs, cut into 1-inch (2.5 cm) pieces (see Note)

1 cup (130 g) peeled, diced carrots, ½-inch (1 cm) dice

1 cup (133 g) diced sweet potatoes, ½-inch (1 cm) cubes

3 tablespoons (45 ml) fresh lemon juice

1 tablespoon (4 g) chopped fresh dill

1 tablespoon (2 g) chopped fresh thyme

1½ teaspoons salt

1 teaspoon black pepper

¼ cup (15 g) chopped fresh parsley

Add the oil to your soup pot over medium-high heat. Once hot, add the onion and celery. Sauté until tender with some browning, 3 to 5 minutes. Add the garlic and sauté for about another minute until the garlic turns a golden color.

Add the stock, chicken, carrots, sweet potatoes, lemon juice, dill, thyme, salt, and black pepper. Bring to a boil over high heat. Cover, reduce the heat to medium, and simmer until the chicken is cooked through, completely opaque and juices run clear, and the sweet potatoes are tender, about 15 minutes.

Stir in the parsley. Taste and add extra salt or black pepper if you like.

Note

If you have a bit more time, keep the chicken breasts whole and simmer until cooked through to a minimum internal temperature of 165°F (74°C), 20 to 25 minutes. Remove to a cutting board, use two forks to shred, and mix back into the soup. I like having shredded chicken in my soup, so I prefer to do it this way when time permits.

Instant Pot Gumbo

YIELD: 8 TO 10 SERVINGS

My take on gumbo doesn't include a traditional roux, but it sure does come bursting with flavor from traditional ingredients like white fish, bell peppers, and shrimp! It's the perfect one-pot meal to add into your rotation that's both paleo and low carb. Serve it with cauliflower rice or regular rice, and it tastes even more fabulous the next day—even cold!

1½ pounds (680 g) wild-caught cod, patted dry and cut into 2-inch (5 cm) chunks

Kosher salt, to taste

Black pepper, to taste

3 tablespoons (10.8 g) Cajun or Creole seasoning, divided

3 tablespoons (45 ml) ghee or avocado oil

4 ribs celery, diced

2 yellow onions, diced

2 green bell peppers, diced

1 can (28 ounces [793 g]) diced tomatoes

1½ cups (350 ml) chicken broth

¼ cup (65 g) tomato paste

3 bay leaves

1½ pounds (680 g) medium or large shrimp, peeled and deveined

Chopped chives or scallion greens, for serving

Sprinkle the cod with salt and black pepper, making sure the pieces are as evenly coated as possible. Sprinkle half the Cajun seasoning evenly onto the fish.

Add the ghee to the Instant Pot and press Sauté. When it reads Hot, add the fish. Sauté until it looks cooked on all sides, about 4 minutes. Use a slotted spoon to transfer the fish to a large plate.

Add the celery, onions, bell peppers, and the remaining Cajun seasoning to the pot and sauté until fragrant, 2 minutes. Press Keep Warm/Cancel.

Add the fish, tomatoes, broth, tomato paste, and bay leaves and give it a nice stir. Put the lid back on the pot and set it to Sealing. Press Manual and set the time for 5 minutes. (The Instant Pot will slowly build up to a high-pressure point and once it reaches that point, the gumbo will cook for 5 minutes.)

Once it's finished cooking, press the Keep Warm/Cancel button. Cautiously change the Sealing valve over to Venting, which will manually release all the pressure.

Once the pressure has been released (this will take a couple of minutes), remove the lid and change the setting to Sauté again. Add the shrimp and cook until the shrimp become opaque and the tails curl, 3 to 4 minutes. Remove the bay leaves and add more salt and black pepper, to taste. Serve topped with chives or scallion greens

Taco Soup

This recipe combines two beloved dishes—tacos and soup—into one meal. It's quick to make, hearty, and freezes wonderfully. This is sure to become a fall and winter staple.

1 tablespoon (15 ml) avocado oil

1 large onion, diced

1 bell pepper, cored and chopped

1 pound (454 g) ground beef

2 tablespoons (12 g) chili powder

1 tablespoon (8 g) ground cumin

1 teaspoon salt

1 teaspoon ground black pepper

1 teaspoon paprika

½ teaspoon garlic powder

½ teaspoon onion powder

1 teaspoon dried oregano

4 cups (946 ml) beef broth

One 14.5-ounce (411 g) can diced tomatoes

One 4-ounce (113 g) can diced green chiles

Heat the avocado oil in a large stockpot over medium heat. Add the onion, bell pepper, and ground beef and cook for 5 minutes.

Add the chili powder, cumin, salt, pepper, paprika, garlic powder, onion powder, oregano, broth, tomatoes, and chiles. Stir well and cook for 15 minutes, or until the veggies are tender.

Ladle into bowls and serve.

Store leftovers, covered, in the refrigerator for up to a week.

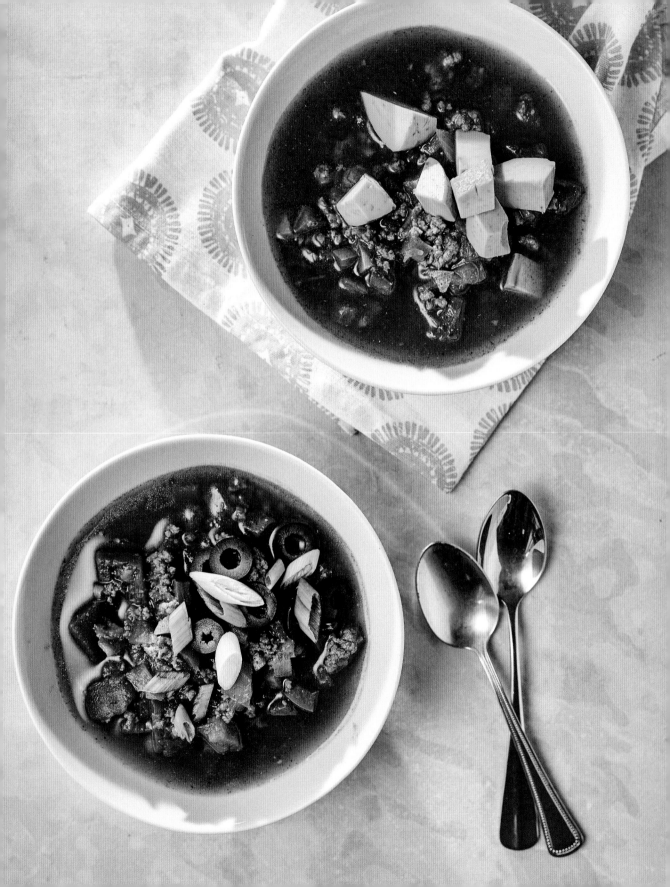

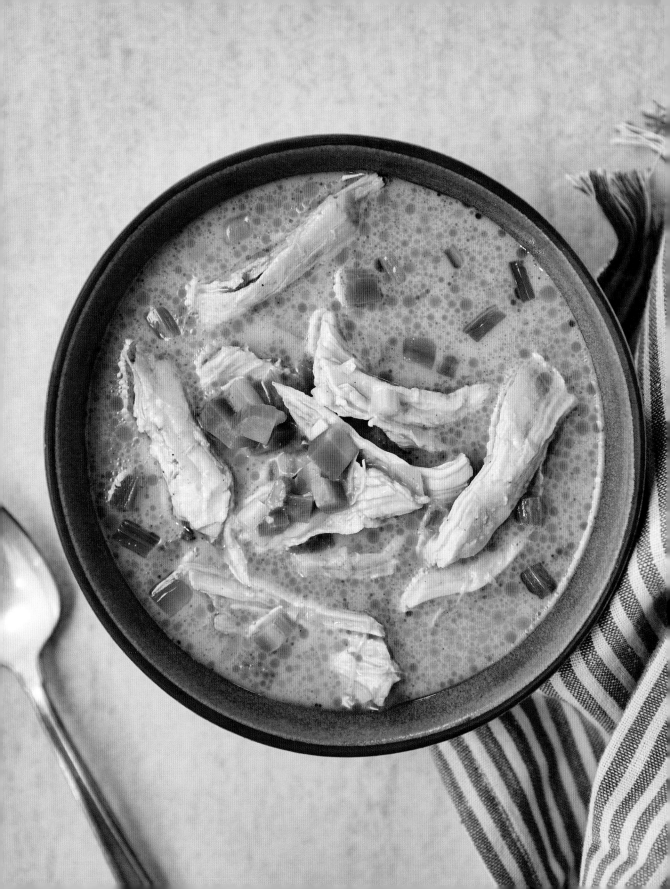

Buffalo Chicken Soup

YIELD: 4 TO 6 SERVINGS

Imagine all the flavors of a buffalo wing, but in soup form. This soup is spiced just right—not too hot—and the ranch dressing gives it a cool creaminess.

2 tablespoons (30 g) ghee

1 cup (120 g) diced celery

3 large carrots, chopped (about 1½ cups [192 g])

1 large onion, diced

3 or 4 cloves garlic, minced

½ teaspoon salt

1–1½ pounds (454–680 g) boneless skinless chicken

¼ cup (60 ml) cayenne pepper sauce, such as Frank's RedHot

4 cups (946 ml) chicken broth

⅓ cup (80 ml) paleo ranch dressing

Heat the ghee in a large stockpot over medium heat. Add the celery, carrots, onion, garlic, and salt. Cook, stirring regularly, for 5 minutes.

Add the chicken, pepper sauce, and broth. Decrease the heat to medium-low, cover, and cook for 15 minutes, or until the chicken is fully cooked through.

Transfer the chicken to a cutting board and chop into bite-size pieces. Return the chicken to the broth and add the ranch dressing. Stir well. Cook over medium heat for 5–10 more minutes, or until fully warmed though.

Ladle into bowls and serve.

Store leftovers, covered, in the refrigerator for up to 6 days.

Chicken Feel-Good Soup

YIELD: 6 TO 8 SERVINGS

This is the soup you need to make when you feel a cold coming on—or you just need a hug in a bowl. The fresh ginger and turmeric are anti-inflammatory foods that will help you heal.

2 tablespoons (30 ml) garlic-infused olive oil

1 tablespoon (15 g) ghee

1 pound (454 g) carrots, sliced into ¼-inch (6 mm)-thick pieces (about 3 cups)

⅔ cup (64 g) chopped green onion

2-inch (5 cm) piece fresh ginger, peeled and grated

1½ teaspoons (9 g) salt

6 cups (1.4 L) water

1 teaspoon turmeric

¼ teaspoon ground black pepper

1½ pounds (680 g) boneless skinless chicken thighs

Heat the olive oil and ghee in a large stockpot over medium heat. Add the carrots, green onion, ginger, and salt. Cook for 3 minutes.

Add the water, turmeric, pepper, and chicken. Bring to a boil over high heat and cook for about 5 minutes, then decrease the heat to medium-low, cover, and cook for 15 minutes.

Remove the chicken and place on a cutting board. Chop into bite-size pieces and return to the soup. Cook for 5 more minutes.

Ladle into bowls and serve immediately.

Store leftovers, covered, in the refrigerator for up to 6 days.

Beef Stew

YIELD: 6 TO 8 SERVINGS

The ingredients are simple, and there is something so nicely familiar about beef stew. This one is just like you remember—hearty, thick, and full of tender beef.

2 tablespoons (30 ml) garlic-infused olive oil, divided

2 pounds (907 g) stew meat or roast cut into 1-inch (3 cm) chunks, divided

1½ teaspoons (9 g) salt, divided

⅓ cup (32 g) chopped green onion

¼ cup (60 ml) coconut aminos

One 14.5-ounce (411 g) can diced tomatoes

3 cups (720 ml) water

2 teaspoons (4 g) chopped fresh thyme

1 cup (120 g) chopped celery

2 cups (300 g) chopped carrots (about 3 carrots)

1 pound (454 g) potatoes, cut into ½-inch (1 cm) chunks

Heat 1 tablespoon (15 ml) of the olive oil in a large stockpot or Dutch oven over medium-high heat. Add 1 pound (454 g) of the meat and ½ teaspoon (3 g) of the salt and cook for about 5 minutes, or until the meat is browned on all sides. Transfer to a plate and repeat with the remaining 1 tablespoon (15 ml) oil, remaining 1 pound (454 g) meat, and ½ teaspoon (3 g) salt.

Return the first batch of beef to the pan. Add the green onion, coconut aminos, tomatoes, water, thyme, and remaining ½ teaspoon (3 g) salt. Decrease the heat to low, cover, and cook, stirring every 30 minutes, for 2 hours.

Add the celery, carrots, and potatoes, cover, and cook for 40–50 minutes, or until all the veggies are tender.

Ladle into bowls and serve immediately.

Store leftovers, covered, in the refrigerator for up to 6 days.

SOUPS

Ham and Potato Soup

YIELD: 4 TO 6 SERVINGS

Tender potatoes and veggies combine with chunks of ham to make this soup irresistible. Blending the potatoes partially makes it amazingly creamy.

1 tablespoon (15 ml) avocado oil

2 cups (223 g) diced celery

1¼ cups (170 g) diced carrots (about 2 medium carrots)

1½ cups (183 g) diced onion (about ½ large onion)

1½ pounds (680 g) potatoes, peeled and chopped into ½-inch (1 cm) pieces (about 4 cups [637 g])

4 cups (946 ml) unsalted chicken broth

1 cup (240 ml) water

1 teaspoon garlic powder

1 teaspoon chopped fresh thyme

¼ teaspoon ground black pepper

1 cup (240 ml) almond milk

2½ ounces kale, chopped (5 cups [71 g])

1 pound (454 g) chopped ham

Salt to taste

Heat the avocado oil in a large stockpot over medium heat. Add the celery, carrots, and onion and cook for 5–7 minutes, or until they start to get tender.

Add the potatoes, broth, water, garlic powder, thyme, and black pepper and bring to a boil over high heat. Decrease the heat to medium-low and cook for 15 minutes, or until the potatoes are tender.

Turn off the heat and add the almond milk. Blend the soup slightly with an immersion blender, making it creamy while still leaving chunks of potatoes.

Add the kale and ham and cook for 5 minutes, or until the kale is wilted. Taste and add salt if needed. Serve warm.

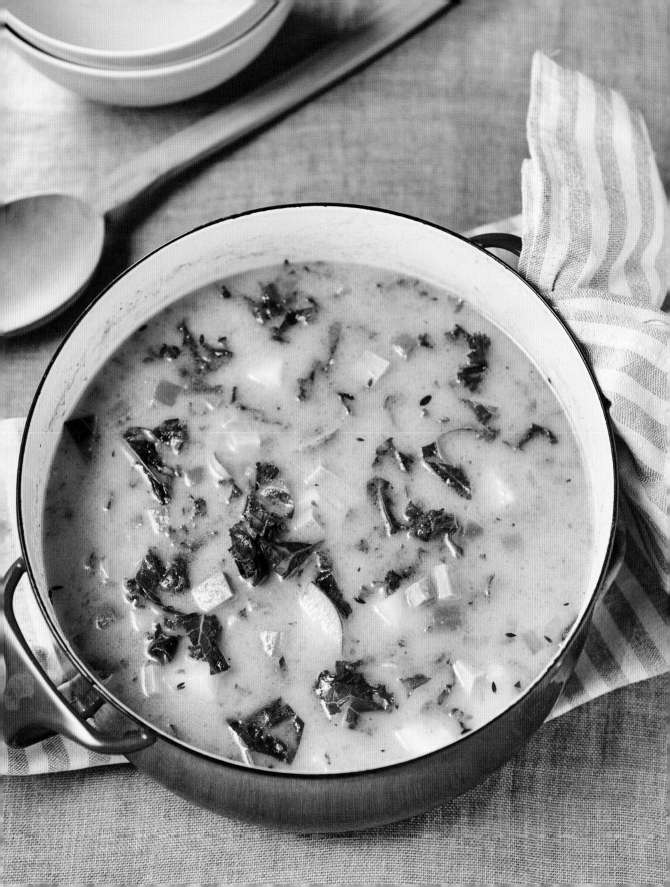

Broccoli Cheese Soup

YIELD: 6 SERVINGS

There is no cheese in this soup, but you won't even be able to tell. The carrots give it the classic look and the lemon juice gives it tang. It's thick, creamy, and loaded with broccoli.

4 cups (364 g) chopped broccoli

2 cups (300 g) chopped carrots (about 3 medium carrots)

1½ pounds (680 g) potatoes, chopped

7 cups (1.7 L) water

1 teaspoon salt

2 tablespoons (30 ml) garlic-infused olive oil

¼ cup (24 g) chopped green onion

2 tablespoons (30 ml) lemon juice

1 cup (240 ml) full-fat coconut milk

1 teaspoon turmeric

Combine the broccoli, carrots, potatoes, water, salt, olive oil, and green onion in a large stockpot and bring to a boil over high heat.

Decrease the heat to medium, cover, and cook for 15–20 minutes, or until the carrots are tender. Remove from the heat. Add the lemon juice, coconut milk, and turmeric.

Blend the soup completely with an immersion blender. Alternatively, transfer batches to a high-powered blender and blend. Be sure to remove the top piece of the lid of the blender and cover with a kitchen towel. This will let the heat release safely.

Ladle into bowls and serve immediately.

Store leftovers, covered, in the refrigerator for up to a week.

CHAPTER FOUR
Main Dishes

Chicken Mole Lettuce Wraps

YIELD: 6 SERVINGS

While a traditional mole sauce can take hours to prepare, you don't need to spend all day over the stove to make this super flavorful and pronounced sauce at home. It's made with pepitas, cashews, raisins, and cacao powder, but don't let the long list of ingredients intimidate you—simply have it ready to go before you begin cooking. You are going to be so impressed with yourself after making this chicken and sauce that's so warm, nourishing, bright, and sassy. Wrap it in some butter lettuce and garnish with the recommended toppings. It's a guaranteed win!

2 tablespoons (30 ml) avocado oil

1 yellow onion, diced

8 cloves garlic, minced

1 can (14.5 ounces [408 g]) fire-roasted crushed tomatoes

Handful of raw cashews

¼ cup (40 g) pepitas, plus more, toasted, for topping

3 tablespoons (45 ml) chicken bone broth or chicken broth

3 tablespoons (21 g) unsweetened raisins

2½ tablespoons (12.5 g) cacao powder

2 tablespoons (15 g) ancho chile powder

1 tablespoon (16 g) tomato paste

1 tablespoon (15 ml) apple cider vinegar

1 teaspoon (2.5 g) paprika

1 teaspoon (6 g) kosher salt, plus more to taste

¼ teaspoon ground cumin

⅛ teaspoon coriander powder

⅛ teaspoon anise powder

Pinch of dried oregano

Pinch of ground cloves

Black pepper, to taste

2 pounds (900 g) boneless, skinless chicken thighs

1 cinnamon stick

Butter lettuce leaves, for serving

Chopped fresh parsley, for topping

Coconut yogurt, for topping

Sliced red onion, for topping

Set the Instant Pot to the Sauté function and add the oil. Once it is hot, add the onion and garlic. Sauté until the onion is soft and the garlic is quite fragrant, 3 to 4 minutes. Press Cancel.

Transfer the onion mixture to the pitcher of a high-speed blender and add the tomatoes, cashews, pepitas, broth, raisins, cacao, ancho chile, tomato paste, vinegar, paprika, salt, cumin, coriander, anise, oregano, cloves, and a few grinds of black pepper. Blend on medium-high speed until creamy throughout.

Add the chicken to the Instant Pot. Pour the mole mixture all over the chicken and add the cinnamon stick. Set the Instant Pot to pressure Cook (Manual) on High, and set the time to 15 minutes.

Once it's done, let the pressure release naturally for 10 minutes. Manually let the pressure out, covering the steam with a kitchen towel. Using two forks, shred and break apart the chicken and mix well into the sauce. Remove the cinnamon stick and discard.

Be sure to taste and adjust the seasoning levels. You will likely need to add more salt to your taste preferences.

Add the chicken mole to butter lettuce leaves and garnish with your desired toppings. Serve warm.

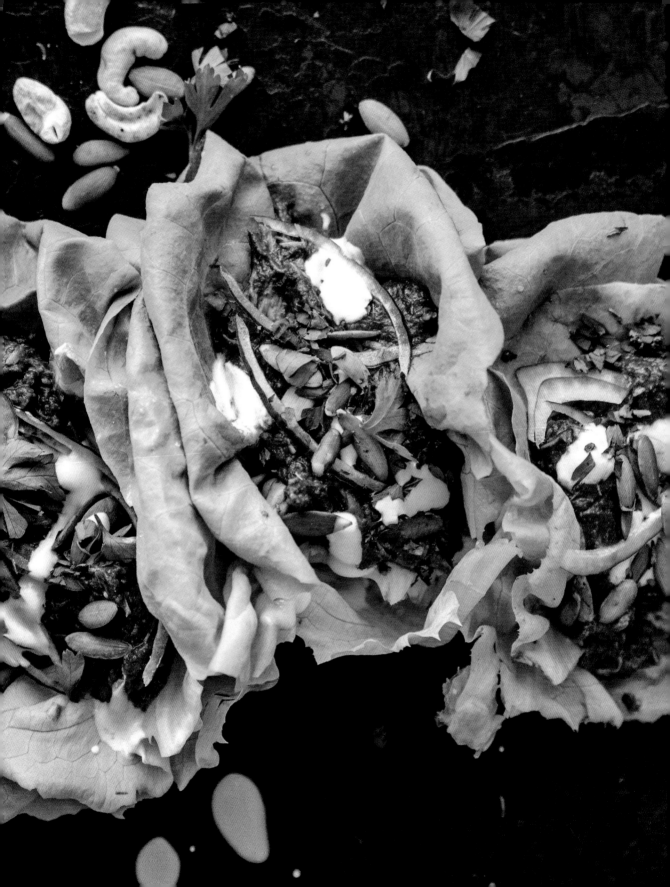

Rice Noodle Shrimp Pad Thai

A rice noodle shrimp pad thai recipe with all of the bold flavors and none of the filler ingredients? Sign me up! The sauce for this dish is absolutely delectable and is made from a short list of ingredients. Use your favorite protein if shrimp aren't your thing, but it's the dry-roasted cashews and scallions that really round out the flavors.

8 ounces (225 g) rice noodles

SAUCE

¼ cup (50 g) coconut sugar

3 tablespoons (45 ml) fish sauce

3 tablespoons (45 ml) coconut aminos

2 tablespoons (30 ml) rice vinegar

2 tablespoons (30 g) cashew butter

1 tablespoon (15 ml) hot sauce

PAD THAI

4 tablespoons (60 ml) avocado oil, divided

1 pound (450 g) large shrimp, peeled, deveined, and patted dry (see Note)

2 large eggs

1 teaspoon (5 ml) filtered water

2 small red bell peppers, julienned

6 cloves garlic, minced

1½ cups (150 g) tightly packed bean sprouts

5 scallions, sliced (reserve some for garnish)

½ cup (75 g) dry-roasted cashews, chopped (reserve some for garnish)

2 limes, cut into wedges

Prepare the rice noodles according to package directions. Drain.

To make the sauce, in a small bowl, whisk together the coconut sugar, fish sauce, coconut aminos, vinegar, cashew butter, and hot sauce until well combined. If your cashew butter isn't creamy, you may see some chunks, and that is fine.

To make the pad thai, heat a large skillet over medium heat and add 2 tablespoons (30 ml) of the oil. When hot (about 2 minutes), add the shrimp in a single layer. Be sure not to over-crowd. Cook until opaque and the tails have curled, 2 to 3 minutes per side, and transfer to a plate or bowl.

In a small bowl, whisk together the eggs and water. Return the skillet to medium heat and add another 1 tablespoon (15 ml) oil. Pour in the eggs and cook undisturbed until no longer runny, about 2 minutes. Transfer the egg to a plate and roughly break apart with a fork.

Add the remaining 1 tablespoon (15 ml) oil to the skillet and return to medium heat. Add the peppers and garlic and cook until slightly soft-ened, stirring occasionally, 4 minutes.

Note

You can use frozen shrimp. Defrost and pat dry before use.

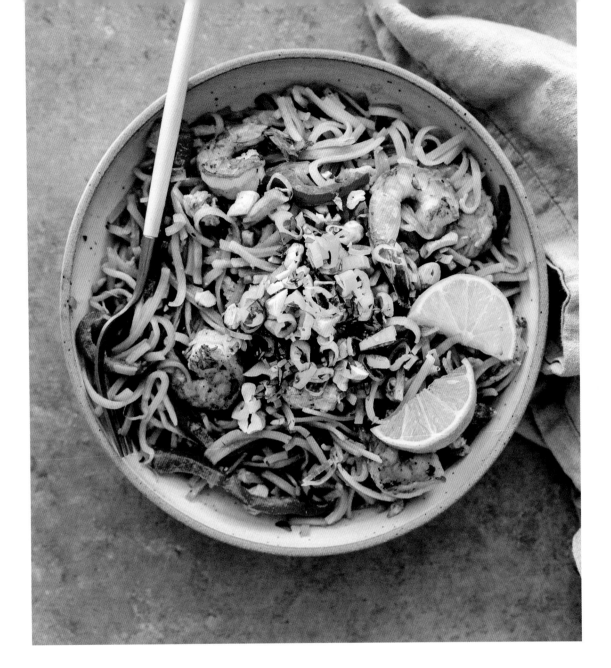

Add the prepared noodles, bean sprouts, scallions (reserving a handful), and cashews (reserving a handful). Cook until the veggies are soft and the flavors have melded together, 3 to 4 minutes. Add the sauce and cook for another 5 minutes, stirring often. Add the shrimp and eggs back to the pan and stir occasionally for 2 more minutes to heat.

Top with more cashews, scallions, and a squeeze of lime before serving.

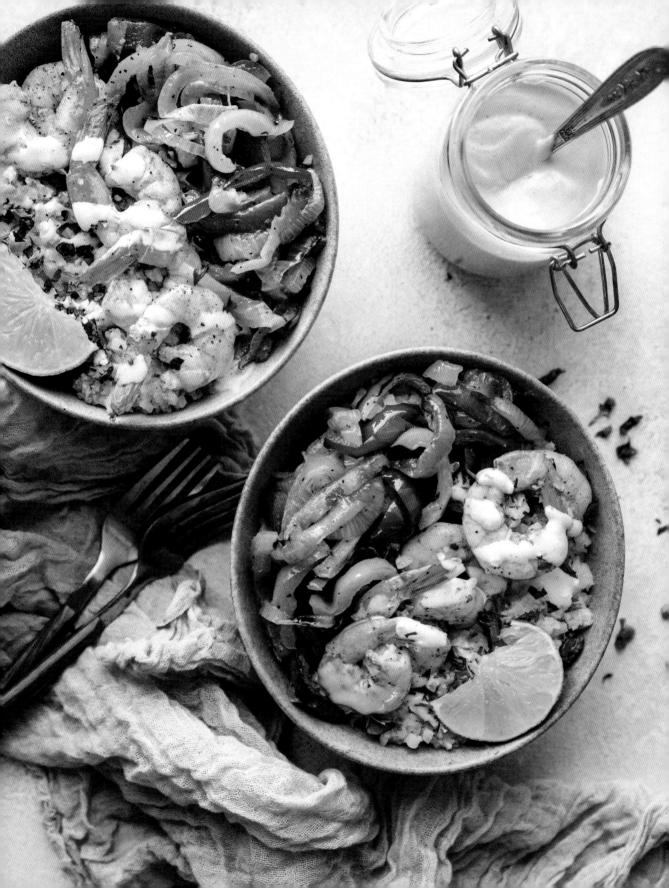

One-Pan Shrimp Fajitas

YIELD: 4 SERVINGS

These shrimp fajitas come together almost magically. The coconut cauliflower rice pairs perfectly with the sizzling shrimp and peppers. There's very little cleanup and lots of flavor—the best one-pan dish!

SHRIMP

3 tablespoons (45 ml) avocado oil

1 lime, juiced

6 cloves garlic, minced

1 teaspoon (6 g) kosher salt

½ teaspoon black pepper

½ teaspoon paprika

½ teaspoon chili powder

½ teaspoon ground cinnamon

Pinch of crushed red pepper flakes

1½ pounds (680 g) extra-large shrimp, peeled, deveined, and tails removed

PEPPERS & ONIONS

3 bell peppers (1 each red, yellow, green), sliced

1 yellow onion, sliced

1½ tablespoons (22 ml) avocado oil

Kosher salt, to taste

Black pepper, to taste

COCONUT CAULIFLOWER RICE

3 cups (450 g) cauliflower rice, cooked

¼ cup (60 ml) full-fat canned coconut milk

2 tablespoons (30 ml) fresh lime juice

1 tablespoon (15 ml) avocado oil

¼ teaspoon kosher salt

⅓ cup (5 g) finely chopped cilantro

Preheat the oven to 450°F (230°C) and adjust the oven rack to the middle position. Line a baking sheet with parchment paper.

To make the shrimp, in a medium bowl, whisk together the oil, lime juice, garlic, salt, black pepper, paprika, chili powder, cinnamon, and red pepper flakes. Add the shrimp and toss thoroughly to completely coat the shrimp. Set aside.

To make the peppers and onions, spread the bell peppers and onion in an even layer on the prepared baking sheet. Add the oil and toss thoroughly to coat everything. Sprinkle with salt and black pepper. Roast until soft throughout, 12 to 15 minutes.

Meanwhile, prepare the rice. In a small bowl, combine the cauliflower, coconut milk, lime juice, oil, and salt. Taste for additional seasoning.

Remove the peppers and onions from the oven and move them to one third of the baking sheet. Add the cauliflower rice to the opposite side (one third of the sheet).

Pour the shrimp and marinade into the center of the baking sheet. Return the pan to the oven and roast until the shrimp have cooked through and look opaque, another 10 to 12 minutes. Remove from the oven and stir the cilantro into the rice. Serve right away.

Clean Paleo Chicken Curry

YIELD: 6 TO 8 SERVINGS

This flavor-forward, easy chicken curry is made with all kinds of spices and nutrient-dense veggies. Try it once and you'll find yourself making this pretty curry time and time again. Serve it with cauliflower rice, rice, or naan bread.

1½ tablespoons (22 ml) ghee or avocado oil, divided

1½ pounds (680 g) boneless, skinless chicken thighs, patted dry and cut into 1-inch (2.5 cm) cubes

Kosher salt, to taste

Black pepper, to taste

¼ cup (60 ml) chicken bone broth or low-sodium chicken broth

1 small yellow onion, diced

¼ cup (60 g) green curry paste

3 cans (13.5 ounces [395 ml]) full-fat coconut milk

1 head cauliflower, cut into small florets

2 cups (300 g) trimmed green beans

2 cups (300 g) diced butternut squash

2 teaspoons (6 g) garlic powder

2 teaspoons (4 g) curry powder

1 teaspoon (1.2 g) crushed red pepper flakes

¾ teaspoon ground ginger

2 teaspoons (4.4 g) turmeric powder

Fresh chopped cilantro, for serving

Heat a high-sided sauté pan with 1 tablespoon (15 ml) of the ghee or oil over medium-high heat. While it is heating up, sprinkle the chicken with salt and black pepper.

Panfry the chicken until lightly brown on all sides, 4 to 5 minutes (it doesn't have to cook through). Using a slotted spoon, transfer the pieces to a bowl and set aside. Discard the excess fat and juice from the pan.

Add the broth and onion to the pan and cook until translucent, 4 to 5 minutes.

Add the remaining ½ tablespoon (7.5 ml) oil to the pan to heat. Add the chicken and the curry paste. Stir until well combined and pour in the coconut milk. Let it just come to a boil and turn down the heat to medium-low.

Add the cauliflower, green beans, squash, garlic powder, curry powder, red pepper flakes, and ginger. Stir to combine and simmer until the vegetables are fork tender, about 12 minutes. Stir in turmeric.

Add salt and black pepper, to taste.

Let the curry simmer until all of the veggies are very tender and the sauce has thickened up a bit, 15 to 20 minutes. Mix in or garnish with fresh cilantro before serving.

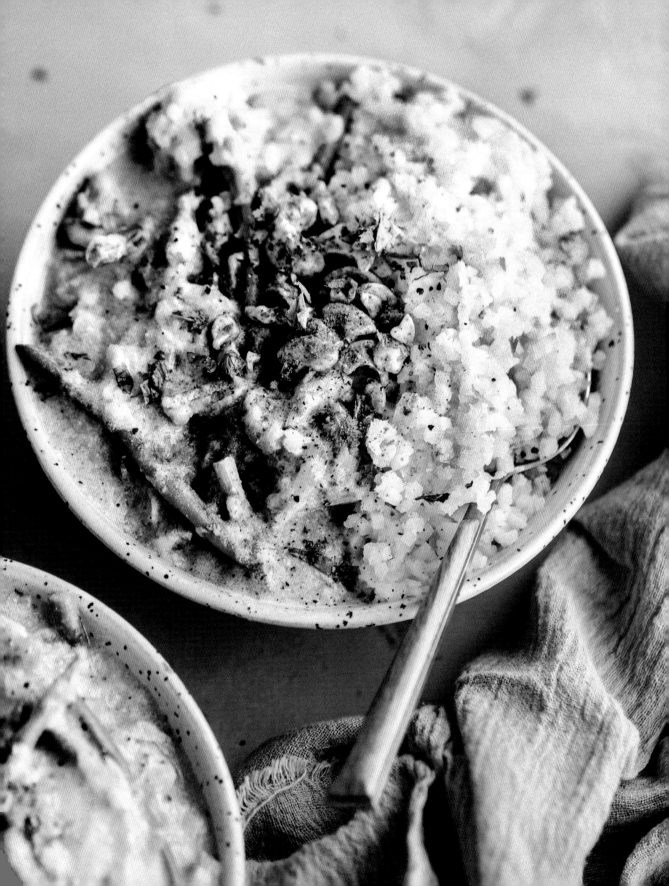

Cauliflower Rice Meatballs

YIELD: 20 MEATBALLS

Is there anything better than adding a nutrient-dense veggie to a meat-centric dish and fooling the crowd? Nope. This is especially true when it comes to getting nutrients in for your kids. These cauliflower rice meatballs, rich with crispy bacon and coconut cream, are paired with a wonderfully zesty sauce. They are absolutely perfect for meal prep and taste delicious when reheated. Serve them over veggie noodles to round out the meal.

MEATBALLS

4 strips bacon, diced

1½ pounds (680 g) grass-fed lean ground beef

1 cup (150 g) cauliflower rice

⅓ cup (50 g) finely diced yellow onion

¼ cup (60 ml) coconut cream (see Note)

1½ teaspoons (9 g) kosher salt

¼ teaspoon ground ginger

1 large egg, whisked

SAUCE

½ cup (120 ml) plus 2 tablespoons (30 ml) coconut aminos

¼ cup (60 ml) plus 1½ tablespoons (22 ml) filtered water, divided

1 tablespoon (15 ml) apple cider vinegar

1½ teaspoons (7.5 ml) extra virgin olive oil

1 teaspoon (2 g) minced fresh ginger

½ teaspoon garlic powder

1 tablespoon (8 g) arrow-root flour

Preheat the oven to 350°F (180°C) and adjust the oven rack to the middle position. Line a baking sheet with parchment paper.

To make the meatballs, in a skillet over medium to medium-high heat, cook the bacon until crispy, about 5 minutes. Transfer to a paper towel–lined plate and let cool.

In a large mixing bowl, combine the ground beef, cauliflower, onion, coconut cream, salt, and ginger. Mix well with your hands, making sure everything is evenly dispersed. Add the egg and mix well again. Finally, add the bacon bits. Mix one last time.

Using a 2-tablespoon (30 ml) cookie scoop, scoop the meatballs and roll them between your palms to create a well-rounded ball. Transfer the meatballs to the prepared baking sheet.

Bake until the middles are just cooked through, 22 to 26 minutes.

Meanwhile, prepare the sauce. In a small saucepan, combine the coconut aminos, ¼ cup (60 ml) of the water, vinegar, oil, ginger, and garlic powder. Set over medium-low heat, stirring constantly, for 10 minutes.

In a small bowl, whisk together the remaining 1½ tablespoons (22 ml) water and arrowroot flour until smooth. Slowly whisk the arrowroot slurry into the sauce, cook for about 1 minute, then remove from the heat.

To serve, toss the meatballs with the sauce or serve them with the sauce on the side.

Note

To make coconut cream, refrigerate a can of full-fat coconut milk overnight and scoop off the top layer that separates. If you can purchase coconut cream, make sure it has 10 to 12 grams of fat.

Beef Bolognese

YIELD: 6 TO 8 SERVINGS

This wonderful beef Bolognese is going to blow your mind. It can all be prepared in one pan, comes together oh so quickly, and has so much flavor, you'd think it had been cooking for days. Be sure to double the batch if you want to save on meal prep. It freezes extremely well and tastes delicious reheated!

8 medium zucchini
(see Note)

2 tablespoons (36 g)
kosher salt, plus more
to taste

6 strips bacon, finely
diced

4 carrots, diced

3 ribs celery, diced

1 yellow onion, diced

8 cloves garlic, minced

2 pounds (900 g)
grass-fed 90 / 10 or
92 / 8 ground beef

2 cans (6 ounces [169 g])
tomato paste

1 cup (240 ml) full-fat
canned coconut milk

1 cup (240 ml) chicken
bone broth or low-sodium
chicken broth

2 teaspoons (6 g) garlic
powder

Black pepper, to taste

Spiralize the zucchini first, as thick or as thin as you'd like. Add the zucchini to a large colander in the sink. Add the salt and massage it into the zucchini. Let it sit for about 20 minutes, as this process will release a lot of moisture. Rinse the zucchini well with cold water and let it drain for another 10 to 15 minutes. Pat it as dry as you can with a kitchen towel and set aside.

Meanwhile, cook the bacon in a large pot over medium-high heat until crunchy, stirring often, about 4 minutes. Transfer the bacon to a paper towel–lined plate.

Lower the heat to medium. Add the carrots, celery, and onion to the pot and cook, stirring occasionally, until the onion appears translucent, about 5 minutes. Add the garlic and cook for another minute or so, until fragrant.

Add the beef and cook, breaking up the pieces, until brown, about 5 minutes. Stir in the tomato paste, coconut milk, broth, and reserved bacon. Bring to a simmer and cook until it thickens, 7 to 10 minutes.

Stir in the garlic powder, along with salt and black pepper, to taste.

Stir in the zucchini noodles and let everything cook together for 4 to 5 minutes. Serve warm.

Note

If you don't have a spiralizer, buy about 2½ pounds (1125 g) precut zoodles.

Baked Polenta with Sausage & Artichoke

YIELD: 4 TO 6 SERVINGS

Are you ready for something that tastes like it came straight out of an authentic Italian restaurant? Well, here it is. This baked polenta dish pretty much gives me lasagna vibes, but it's actually super light. It's the perfect weeknight meal and tastes delicious when reheated as leftovers.

2 tablespoons (30 ml) avocado oil

½ white onion, diced large

1 pound (450 g) Italian sausage, casings removed

4 cloves garlic, minced

1 cup (150 g) artichoke hearts in water, drained and coarsely chopped

Kosher salt, to taste

Black pepper, to taste

1½ pounds (680 g) polenta, prepared in a tube, sliced into ½-inch (1.3 cm) rounds

⅓ cup (80 ml) chicken broth

1½ cups (350 ml) red sauce (marinara sauce)

¼ cup (22 g) grated Parmesan cheese (optional)

¼ cup (12.5 g) fresh parsley, chopped

Preheat the oven to 400°F (200°C) and adjust the oven rack to the middle position.

In a large skillet over medium heat, add the oil. After 1 minute, add the onion. Cook until soft, stirring frequently, about 5 minutes.

Add the sausage and cook, while breaking up the meat with a wooden spoon, until browned, 7 to 8 minutes. Add the garlic and cook for about 1 minute, stirring frequently, until fragrant.

Remove the skillet from the heat and stir in the artichoke hearts and a big pinch of salt and pepper.

Transfer the mixture to a 2-quart (2 L) baking dish and nestle the polenta rounds in it. Pour the broth evenly on top of the dish. Cover with the red sauce and cheese, if using.

Bake until the polenta is glistening and the cheese has melted, 20 to 25 minutes. Sprinkle with the parsley and serve warm.

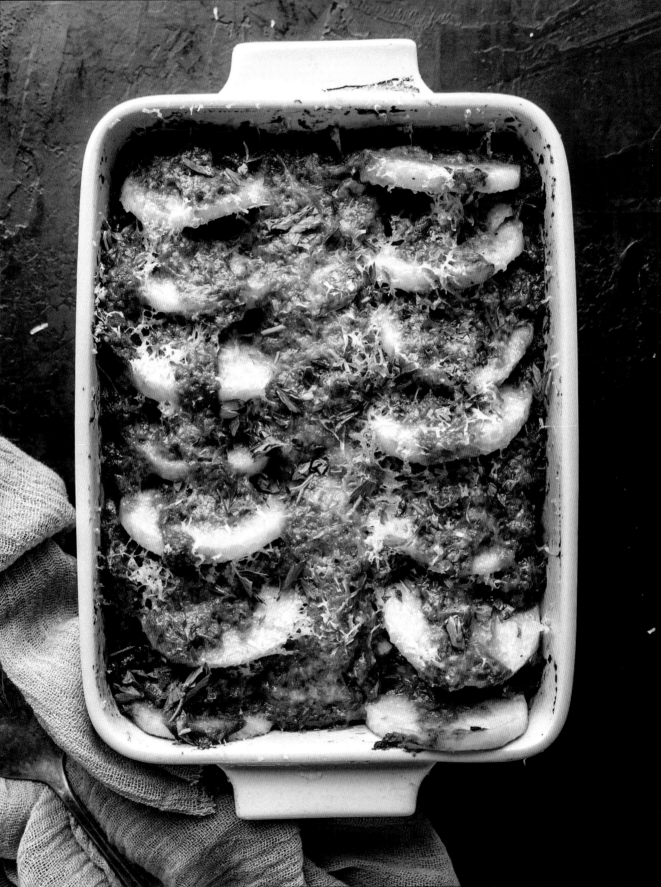

Best Curry Meatballs

YIELD: 24 MEATBALLS

These meatballs are the perfect addition to your weekly meal plan. Bring them with you to lunch atop a big and hearty salad, or enjoy them with a large bowl of cauliflower rice for dinner. Be sure to double up on the delicious, creamy sauce, too—you are going to wish you had extra to slather over all kinds of dinners throughout the week.

MEATBALLS

1 cup (150 g) coarsely chopped carrots

½ cup (75 g) cooked cauliflower rice

½ red onion, coarsely chopped

3 tablespoons (7.5 g) chopped fresh basil, plus more for garnish

6 cloves garlic

1½ limes, juiced

2 tablespoons (30 ml) coconut aminos

1 tablespoon (7 g) flax-seed meal

1½ teaspoons (1.8 g) ground ginger

1 teaspoon (2.5 g) ground cumin

½ teaspoon crushed red pepper flakes, plus more for garnish

½ teaspoon kosher salt

½ teaspoon black pepper

Splash of fish sauce

2 pounds (900 g) grass-fed 90/10 ground beef

CURRY SAUCE

1 can (13.5 ounces [380 ml]) full-fat coconut milk

3 tablespoons (45 g) cashew butter or almond butter

2 heaping tablespoons (30 g) red curry paste

2 limes, juiced

2 teaspoons (6 g) minced garlic

½ teaspoon ground ginger

2 tablespoons (16 g) arrowroot flour, whisked with 2 tablespoons (30 ml) filtered water (optional)

Preheat the oven to 375°F (190°C) and adjust the oven rack to the middle position. Line a baking sheet with parchment paper.

To make the meatballs, place the carrots, cauliflower rice, onion, basil, garlic, lime juice, coconut aminos, flax, ginger, cumin, red pepper flakes, salt, black pepper, and fish sauce in the bowl of a food processor. Pulse for 30 seconds or so until mixed well. Do not overprocess, or the mixture will become mushy! Add the beef and process a few more times.

Roll the mixture into 1½ to 2-inch (4 to 5 cm) balls and place them on the prepared baking sheet.

Bake for 20 minutes and rotate the sheet 180 degrees. Bake for another 10 to 15 minutes, until the meatballs have reached your desired doneness. I like mine cooked to a medium doneness, so I pull them out after 30 minutes total.

While the meatballs finish baking, prepare the sauce. In a medium saucepan, heat the coconut milk until it begins to simmer. Add the nut butter, curry paste, lime juice, garlic, and ginger and whisk well. Bring to a low boil, then turn the heat down to low. Let simmer and thicken for 10 to 15 minutes. If you like your sauce a bit thicker, you can add the optional arrowroot mixture.

Serve the meatballs covered with the curry sauce and garnished with fresh basil and red pepper flakes, if desired.

Tuscan Shrimp

YIELD: 4 TO 5 SERVINGS

This quick shrimp dish brings home the flavors of Tuscany: sun-dried tomatoes, spinach, and a delectable cream sauce. Serve with a beautiful side salad to make a complete meal.

1 tablespoon (14 g) ghee

1½ pounds (680 g) jumbo peeled and deveined shrimp

1 cup (240 ml) compliant chicken broth

⅓ cup (80 ml) canned unsweetened coconut milk

1½ tablespoons (9 g) arrowroot powder or tapioca flour dissolved in 2 tablespoons (30 ml) water (see Note)

2 cups (60 g) baby spinach

¼ cup (27 g) no-sugar-added whole sun-dried tomatoes in olive oil

1 tablespoon (15 ml) lemon juice

Sea salt and black pepper to taste

Chopped fresh parsley, for garnish

1 bag (12 ounces [336 g]) cauliflower rice, steamed (optional)

Heat the ghee in a large skillet over medium heat until the ghee starts to sizzle. Add the shrimp and cook until pink or opaque and the tails curl, 3 to 4 minutes, flipping once. Remove the shrimp to a plate and set aside.

Add the broth and coconut milk to the skillet and stir together.

Add the arrowroot mixture and whisk until thickened, 2 to 3 minutes.

Add the spinach, tomatoes, and lemon juice. Stir together and add salt and pepper to taste.

Return the shrimp to the skillet and simmer over low heat for 2 minutes to combine and warm through.

Sprinkle with the parsley and serve over cauliflower rice or mash, if desired.

Note

The gravy won't be as thick as when made with regular flour. It is the consistency of a thicker soup. Feel free to add less broth to make it thicker, or experiment with adding a little more tapioca flour. Remember that it will begin to thicken as it heats.

Spinach-Artichoke Chicken

YIELD: 4 SERVINGS

One-skillet dishes save lives because cleanup is a breeze. This skillet dinner can be ready in 30 minutes or less by using an electric pressure cooker to cook the spaghetti squash.

1 small (3- to 4-pound [1.3 to 1.8 kg]) spaghetti squash

Olive oil, for the squash

1 tablespoon (14 g) ghee

1 pound (454 g) boneless, skinless chicken breasts

1 can (4 ounces [112 g]) sliced mushrooms, drained

1 cup (30 g) baby spinach

4 artichoke hearts, quartered

1 clove garlic, minced

1 cup (240 ml) compliant chicken broth

½ cup (120 ml) canned unsweetened coconut milk

1 lemon, ½ juiced, ½ sliced for garnish

1½ tablespoons (9 g) tapioca flour

½ teaspoon sea salt

¼ teaspoon black pepper

¼ teaspoon onion powder

Chopped fresh parsley, for garnish

Cooking spaghetti squash in the oven

Heat the oven to 400°F (200°C or gas mark 6). Slice the squash in half lengthwise and scoop out the seeds. Drizzle the halves with olive oil and sprinkle with sea salt. Place cut-side down on a baking sheet and roast until tender, 45 to 50 minutes. Let cool slightly, then use a fork to shred the squash flesh.

Cooking spaghetti squash in the electric pressure cooker

Pierce the squash all over with a paring knife. Place a trivet or steamer basket in the bottom of the electric pressure cooker, set the squash on top, and add 1 cup (240 ml) water to the bottom. Cook on high pressure for 15 minutes. Use instant release to release the cooker's pressure. Remove the squash and let cool slightly. Halve lengthwise, drizzle with olive oil, and sprinkle with salt. Shred the squash flesh with a fork.

Spinach-Artichoke Chicken

Prepare the spaghetti squash.

Heat the ghee in a large skillet over medium-high heat until it sizzles.

Add the chicken and cook until the internal temperature reaches 160°F (71°C), about 5 minutes on each side. Remove the chicken to a cutting board, let cool slightly, and then chop.

To the hot skillet, add the mushrooms, spinach, artichoke hearts, and garlic. Cook until heated through and the spinach wilts, 2 to 3 minutes. Add the chicken back to the skillet, stirring to combine.

Stir in the spaghetti squash and mix together.

In a medium bowl, whisk together the broth, coconut milk, lemon juice, tapioca flour, salt, black pepper, and onion powder.

Pour the broth mixture into the skillet and stir to combine well.

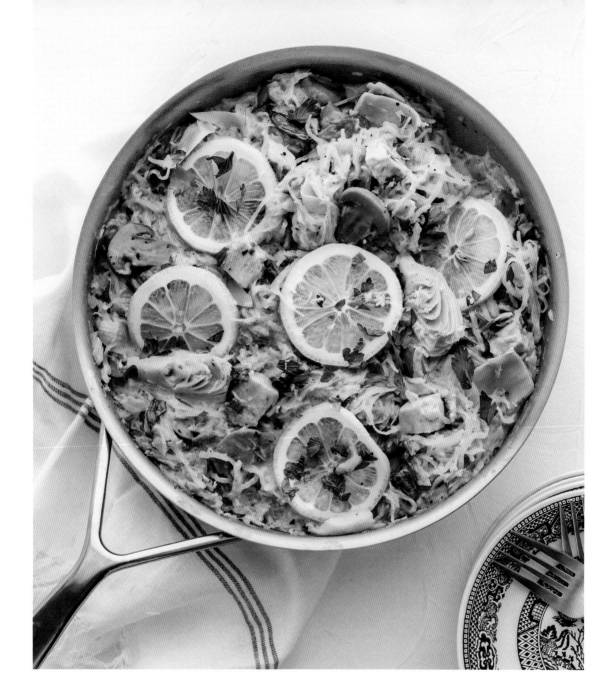

Reduce the heat to low and simmer until the sauce begins to thicken, about 3 minutes.

Garnish with the parsley and lemon slices before serving. For a cheesy texture and taste, sprinkle the top of this skillet with a few shakes of nutritional yeast.

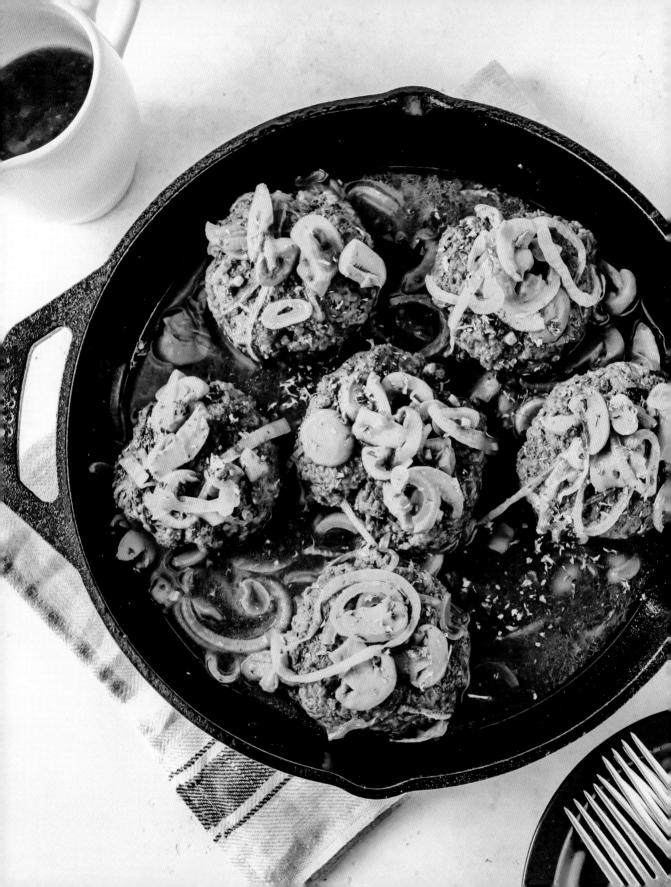

Hamburger Steaks

YIELD: 6 SERVINGS

Nothing says "family dinner" like skillet hamburger steaks. These juicy burger patties bathe in a broth that is packed with garlic, sautéed onions, and mushrooms.

2 pounds (910 g) 90/10 ground beef

¾ teaspoon sea salt, divided

½ teaspoon black pepper, divided

1 tablespoon (15 ml) olive oil

1 teaspoon ghee

1 small onion, sliced

1 can (8 ounces [224 g]) sliced mushrooms, drained

2 cups (480 ml) compliant beef broth

¼ teaspoon onion powder

¼ teaspoon garlic powder

1 teaspoon coarsely chopped fresh parsley

Gently form the ground beef into 6 hamburger patties. Indent the middle of each patty with your thumb to help keep the form while cooking. Sprinkle the patties on both sides with ½ teaspoon of the salt and ¼ teaspoon of the pepper.

Heat the olive oil in a large skillet over medium-high heat. Add the patties, leaving space between them.

Cook the patties until the desired doneness, or when the internal temperature reaches 160°F (71°C), 5 to 6 minutes per side. Remove the burgers to a plate.

Add the ghee to the skillet, along with the sliced onion and mushrooms. Stir together and cook until the onion softens, 3 to 4 minutes.

Add the broth, onion powder, garlic powder, remaining ¼ teaspoon salt, and remaining ¼ teaspoon pepper. Cook until heated through, 1 to 2 minutes.

Return the hamburger patties to the skillet and use a spoon to cover them with the sauce and veggies.

Sprinkle with the parsley before serving.

Note

I did not use a thickening agent with this dish because the broth is so good without it. If you want the broth to be thick, add 1½ tablespoons (9 g) tapioca flour dissolved in 2 tablespoons (30 ml) water to the broth mixture in step 5.

Creamy Mushroom Bacon Chicken Thighs

YIELD: 4 TO 5 SERVINGS

These perfect one-skillet chicken thighs are drenched in a creamy mushroom-garlic sauce and topped with crisp bacon. This meal can be ready in 15 minutes or less.

1 tablespoon (15 ml) olive oil

4 or 5 large bone-in, skin-on chicken thighs

1 teaspoon sea salt

½ teaspoon black pepper

½ teaspoon garlic powder

1 tablespoon (14 g) ghee

2 cans (4 ounces [112 g]) mushrooms, drained

½ large sweet onion, thinly sliced

2 cloves garlic, minced

1½ cups (360 ml) compliant chicken broth

2 tablespoons (30 ml) canned unsweetened coconut milk

½ teaspoon onion powder

¼ teaspoon sea salt (more to taste)

¼ teaspoon black pepper

1½ tablespoons (9 g) tapioca flour dissolved in 2 tablespoons (30 ml) water

2 pieces cooked compliant bacon, chopped

3 tablespoons (12 g) chopped fresh parsley

Heat the olive oil in a large skillet over medium-high heat.

Pat each chicken thigh dry with a paper towel, then coat each thigh with a mixture of the salt, pepper, and garlic powder.

Add the chicken to the skillet and cook until the juices run clear and the internal temperature is 160°F (71°C), 7 to 8 minutes on each side.

Remove the chicken to a plate but keep the drippings in the skillet.

Add the ghee and when it sizzles, add the mushrooms, onion, and garlic.

Cook until the onion browns, 2 to 3 minutes. Then add the broth, coconut milk, onion powder, salt, and pepper. Stir until heated through.

Turn the heat to low. Add the tapioca mixture and whisk until thickened. (It will begin to thicken as it heats up; it won't happen instantly.)

Once thick, add the chicken thighs back to the gravy and cook for another 3 to 4 minutes.

Serve topped with crispy bacon and fresh parsley for garnish.

Note

For keto, use ¼ teaspoon xanthan gum or 1½ tablespoons (14 g) of gelatin to thicken.

Halibut in Tomato Cream Sauce

YIELD: 4 SERVINGS

Layers of cauliflower rice, tomatoes, butternut squash, and halibut are topped with an easy tomato cream sauce for a dinner that looks as good as it tastes.

TOMATO CREAM SAUCE

1 can (28 ounces, or 785 g) crushed tomatoes

¾ cup (175 ml) canned unsweetened coconut milk, stirred

1½ teaspoons minced garlic

1 teaspoon salt

1 teaspoon dried oregano

1 teaspoon dried basil

½ teaspoon crushed red pepper flakes

½ teaspoon black pepper

HALIBUT & VEGGIES

2 packages (10 ounces, or 280 g, each) cauliflower rice, steamed

2 medium tomatoes, sliced ¼-inch (6 mm) thick

2 cups (280 g) diced butternut squash, 1-inch (2.5 cm) cubes (see Note)

4 halibut fillets (6 ounces, or 170 g, each)

½ teaspoon salt

4 or 5 fresh basil leaves, chopped

Preheat the oven to 425°F (220°C, or gas mark 7).

Make the Tomato Cream Sauce: In a large bowl, combine the crushed tomatoes, coconut milk, garlic, salt, oregano, basil, red pepper flakes, and black pepper. Set aside.

Make the Halibut & Veggies: Spread the steamed cauliflower rice in the bottom of a 9 x 13-inch (23 x 33 cm) baking dish. Layer the tomatoes on top of the cauliflower and spread half of the Tomato Cream Sauce over the tomatoes. Layer the squash next and top with the halibut. Sprinkle the halibut with the salt and then spread the remaining sauce over everything.

Bake until the fish is opaque and flakes easily with a fork and the squash is tender, about 20 minutes. Garnish with the fresh basil before serving.

Note

Cut the butternut squash into cubes ¾ to 1 inch (2 to 2.5 cm) big. Some grocery stores carry pre-chopped squash in this very size. It's a huge time-saver!

Quick Pepper Steak Stir-Fry

YIELD: 4 SERVINGS

This Asian-inspired pepper steak stir-fry is perfect for when you're craving Chinese takeout—and it's about as quick to make as it would be to order. Serve it over cauliflower rice to make this a complete takeout copycat meal.

1 tablespoon (15 ml) olive oil

1 red bell pepper, cut into 1-inch (2.5 cm) squares

1 green bell pepper, cut into 1-inch (2.5 cm) squares

1½ pounds (680 g) flank steak, thinly sliced against the grain into ½ by 4-inch (1.3 by 10 cm) strips

Sea salt and black pepper

2 cloves garlic, minced

½ cup (120 ml) coconut aminos

1½ tablespoons (23 ml) rice wine vinegar

1 tablespoon (15 ml) sesame oil

1 teaspoon tapioca flour

½ teaspoon ground ginger

¼ teaspoon onion powder

¼ teaspoon black pepper

Sliced scallions, for garnish

Sesame seeds, for garnish

Heat the olive oil in a large skillet over medium-high heat.

Add the bell peppers and cook until tender, 3 to 4 minutes. Remove to a dish and set aside.

Sprinkle the steak with salt and pepper. Add to the skillet, along with the garlic. Cook, stirring frequently, until the steak is tender, about 6 minutes.

Meanwhile, in a small bowl, whisk together the coconut aminos, rice wine vinegar, sesame oil, tapioca, ginger, onion powder, and black pepper.

Add the sauce and the bell peppers to the skillet. Simmer until the sauce thickens, 3 minutes.

Divide among bowls and garnish with scallions and sesame seeds.

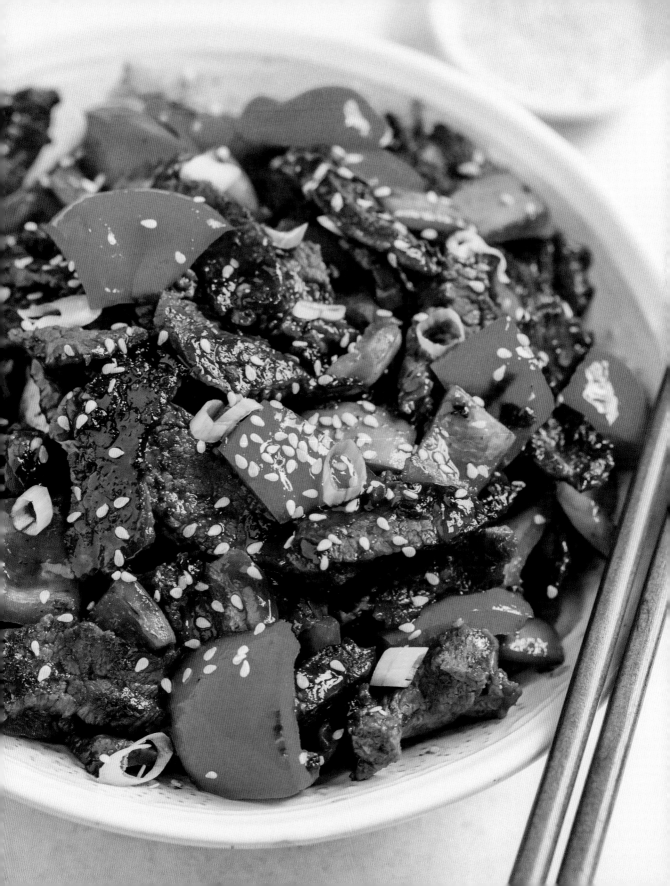

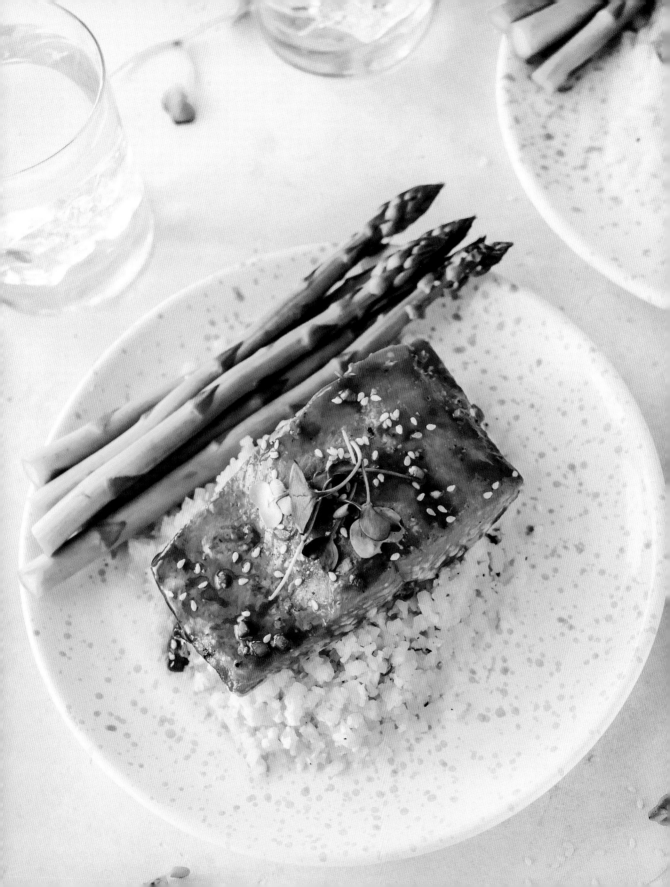

Teriyaki Salmon

YIELD: 4 SERVINGS

This baked salmon is tender and flavorful and takes only 15 minutes to make. It can serve as the perfect healthy weeknight meal.

TERIYAKI SAUCE

¾ cup (180 ml) coconut aminos

¼ cup (60 ml) fresh squeezed orange juice

2 tablespoons (30 ml) pineapple juice

2 tablespoons (30 ml) sesame oil

1 clove garlic, minced

¼ teaspoon ground ginger

1 tablespoon (6 g) tapioca flour dissolved in 1½ tablespoons (23 ml) water

SALMON

4 salmon fillets (4 ounces [112 g] each)

1 tablespoon (15 ml) olive oil

2 tablespoons (30 g) coarse sea salt

1 bunch asparagus, trimmed

Chopped scallions, for garnish

Sesame seeds, for garnish

Microgreens, for garnish

4 cups (560 g) cauliflower rice, cooked

Teriyaki sauce

In a small saucepan over medium heat, whisk together the coconut aminos, orange juice, pineapple juice, sesame oil, garlic, and ginger.

Once the mixture comes to a slow boil, add the tapioca mixture and whisk to combine.

Turn the heat to low. As it continues to heat, the sauce will become thicker.

Once thick, remove from the heat.

Salmon

Preheat the oven to 350°F (180°C or gas mark 4) and line a baking sheet with aluminum foil.

Place the salmon on the baking sheet and drizzle the olive oil on each fillet.

Bake until the salmon is sizzling, 10 minutes.

Meanwhile, bring 8 cups (2 L) water and the salt to a boil in a large saucepan. Prepare a large bowl with ice and water. Add the asparagus to the saucepan and boil until crisp-tender, 3 minutes. Remove the asparagus to the ice water and let cool for 1 minute.

Remove the salmon from the oven and brush the teriyaki sauce on each fillet.

Garnish with the scallions, sesame seeds, and microgreens.

Serve with the asparagus and cauliflower rice.

Shredded Pork

YIELD: 8 TO 10 SERVINGS

This easy shredded pork will make you forget about that BBQ joint down the street. The recipe has minimal ingredients but maximum flavor. Make a big batch at the beginning of the week and use it for multiple meals throughout the week.

4 pounds (1.8 kg) bone-less pork shoulder

1 teaspoon garlic powder

1 teaspoon sea salt

1 teaspoon black pepper

½ cup (120 ml) water

Juice of ½ lime (optional)

Note

This dish is great to make in bulk and serve in different ways throughout the week, from nachos to salads.

Electric pressure cooker version

Slice the pork into 4 equal pieces and sprinkle with the garlic powder, salt, and pepper.

Place the water in the bottom of the electric pressure cooker and then add the pork.

Lock the lid and seal the top vent. Press MANUAL and set for 45 minutes.

Allow the pot to naturally release the steam.

Remove the pork to a large cutting board and shred with two forks.

Add the pork along with the remaining juices from the pot and the lime juice, if using, to a large serving bowl.

Store any leftovers in an airtight container along with the juices. Will keep for up to a week in the fridge.

Slow cooker version

Place the pork on a cutting board and cover the entire piece with the garlic powder, salt, and pepper.

Place the water in the bottom of the slow cooker and then add the pork.

Cover and cook until the internal temperature reaches 190°F (88°C), on LOW for 7 to 8 hours.

Remove the pork to a large cutting board and shred with two forks.

Add the pork along with the remaining juices from the pot and the lime juice, if using, to a large serving bowl.

Salsa Verde Chicken

YIELD: 6 TO 8 SERVINGS

Meal prep has never been easier (or yummier) than with this super easy salsa verde chicken. It's so versatile, it can leave you building different delicious meals throughout the week. Add it to a lettuce wrap, on top of salads, or have it with cauliflower rice and veggies.

2 to 3 teaspoons olive oil

½ cup (80 g) chopped yellow onion

1 jar (16 ounces [454 g]) compliant, no-sugar-added salsa verde

1 can (14 ounces [392 g]) diced tomatoes, drained

Juice of ½ lime

6 chicken breasts (1½ pounds [680 g] total)

1 teaspoon ghee

1 teaspoon ground cumin

1 teaspoon garlic powder

1 teaspoon sea salt

½ teaspoon black pepper

½ teaspoon chili powder

Note

Store the shredded chicken in the juices in an airtight container in the refrigerator for up to 5 days, or in the freezer for up to 3 months.

Electric pressure cooker version

Set the electric pressure cooker to SAUTÉ and allow time for it to heat up.

Add 3 teaspoons olive oil and the onion to the pot. Sauté until tender, a minute or two.

Add the salsa verde, tomatoes, and lime juice. Stir to combine.

Submerge the chicken breasts in the liquid. Add the ghee, cumin, garlic powder, salt, pepper, and chili powder.

Lock the lid and seal the top vent.

Cook on HIGH pressure for 10 minutes, then quick release the steam until the pin drops.

Shred the chicken in the pot using two forks or an electric mixer (see Note).

Mix the shredded chicken with the juices in the pot before serving.

Slow cooker version

Heat a small skillet with 2 teaspoons olive oil over medium-high heat. Add the onion and cook until tender, 3 minutes. Set aside.

Place the chicken breasts in the slow cooker.

Top with the salsa verde, tomatoes, cooked onion, lime juice, ghee, cumin, garlic powder, salt, pepper, and chili powder.

Cover and cook until the chicken is tender, on HIGH for 3 to 4 hours or on LOW for 7 to 8 hours.

Shred the chicken in the pot using two forks or an electric mixer (see Note).

Mix the shredded chicken with the juices in the pot before serving.

Easy Cashew Chicken

YIELD: 4 SERVINGS

Serve up this easy chicken dish on any busy weeknight! Chicken, cashews, broccoli, red bell pepper, and the tastiest 4-ingredient sauce ever—what's not to love? It has all the flavor you want in exceptional takeout, but it's better for you. Feel free to swap out the chicken for pork tenderloin, if that's what you have on hand.

4-INGREDIENT SAUCE

½ cup (120 ml) coconut aminos

1 tablespoon (15 ml) rice or apple cider vinegar

1 tablespoon (10 g) minced garlic

¼ to ½ teaspoon crushed red pepper flakes

CASHEW CHICKEN & VEGGIES

1½ pounds (680 g) boneless, skinless chicken breast, cut into 1-inch (2.5 cm) pieces

12 ounces (340 g) broccoli florets, large florets cut in half or thirds

1 red bell pepper, sliced into strips

Salt and black pepper to taste

2 tablespoons (28 ml) extra-virgin olive oil

¾ cup (105 g) roasted cashews, salted or unsalted

Preheat the oven to 425°F (220°C, or gas mark 7).

Make the 4-Ingredient Sauce: In a bowl, whisk together the coconut aminos, vinegar, garlic, and red pepper flakes (use more for spicier flavor!). Set aside.

Make the Cashew Chicken & Veggies: Spread the chicken in a single layer on one side of a 12 x 17-inch (30 x 43 cm) baking sheet.

Add the broccoli in a single layer beside your chicken.

Spread the bell pepper in a single layer beside the broccoli.

Sprinkle salt and black pepper over everything. Drizzle the oil over the broccoli and bell pepper. Drizzle half the sauce over the chicken. (Save the other half for later.) Bake for 10 minutes.

Remove from the oven and separate the chicken if it's sticking together. Make room for the cashews and add directly to the pan. Bake for 5 additional minutes.

Remove from the oven and make sure your chicken is cooked through, completely opaque and juices run clear. Layer the broccoli, bell pepper, chicken, and cashews in bowls or on plates. Drizzle the remaining sauce on top just before serving.

Notes

In most recipes, I mention using parchment paper on your baking sheet. I don't use any for this particular recipe, but you're welcome to if you'd like to further minimize cleanup.

I love to serve this recipe over steamed cauliflower rice to create larger portion sizes and add an extra boost of veggies!

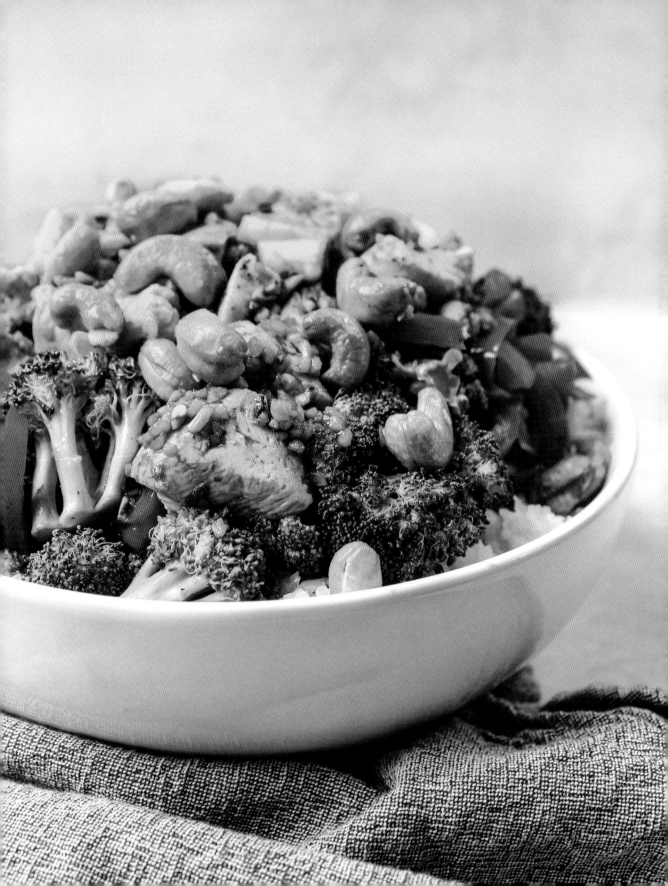

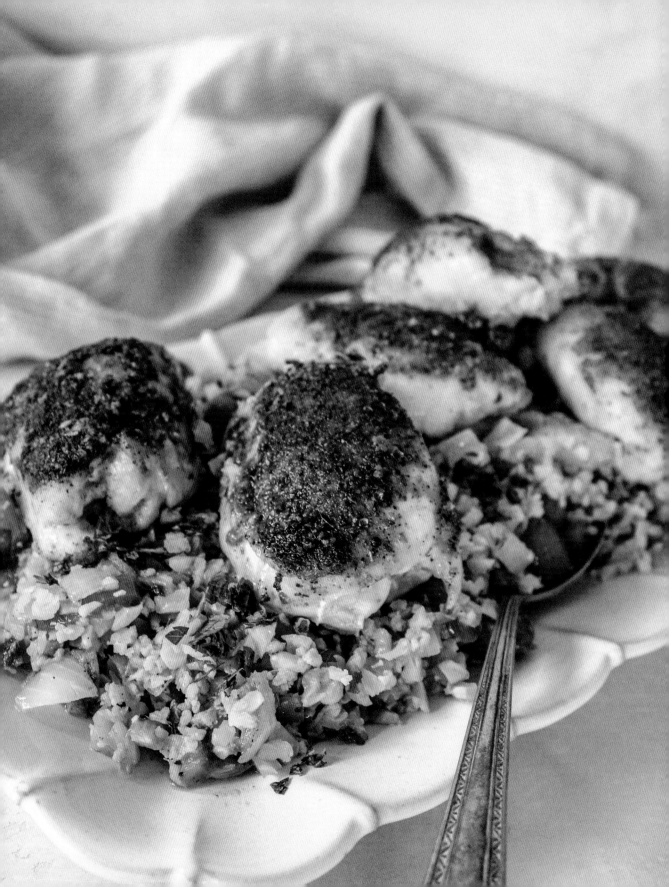

Arroz con Pollo

YIELD 4 SERVINGS

This fun and light twist on a classic Spanish chicken dish is so flavorful you are going to want to make it again and again. Juicy chicken thighs coated in a homemade adobo seasoning bake with veggie-packed cauliflower rice for a bold sheet-pan meal.

ADOBO SEASONING

1½ teaspoons salt

1 teaspoon paprika

½ teaspoon dried oregano

½ teaspoon black pepper

¼ teaspoon chili powder

¼ teaspoon ground cumin

¼ teaspoon onion powder

¼ teaspoon garlic powder

CHICKEN

1½ to 2 pounds (680 to 900 g) boneless, skinless chicken thighs

1 tablespoon (15 ml) extra-virgin olive oil

CAULIFLOWER RICE

3 cups (12 ounces, or 340 g) cauliflower rice

1 cup (180 g) halved grape tomatoes

½ green bell pepper, diced into ½-inch (1 cm) pieces

½ red bell pepper, diced into ½-inch (1 cm) pieces

½ white or yellow onion, diced into ½-inch (1 cm) pieces

1 tablespoon (15 ml) extra-virgin olive oil

Small handful of fresh parsley, chopped

Preheat the oven to 425°F (220°C, or gas mark 7).

Make the Adobo Seasoning: In a small bowl, combine the salt, paprika, oregano, black pepper, chili powder, cumin, onion powder, and garlic powder. Set aside.

Make the Chicken: Pat the chicken thighs dry. Rub the oil on the chicken, focusing most of it on the top. Press all but 1 teaspoon of the Adobo Seasoning onto the top of your chicken. Place the chicken on one side of a 12 x 17-inch (30 x 43 cm) sheet pan.

Make the Cauliflower Rice: Spread the cauliflower rice on the empty side of your sheet pan. Add the tomatoes, bell peppers, and onion to the cauliflower. Drizzle the oil over the veggies and sprinkle on another 1 teaspoon Adobo Seasoning.

Bake for 20 minutes. This cooks fairly quickly since we're using boneless thighs. To crisp the top of the chicken a bit, broil on high for 2 to 3 minutes after the baking time finishes.

Remove from the oven and cover the sheet pan with aluminum foil. Let the chicken rest for 10 minutes so that it's tender and completely cooked through to a minimum internal temperature of 165°F (74°C). Top the Cauliflower Rice with the parsley before serving.

Lemon Garlic Mahi Mahi with Carrots

YIELD: 4 SERVINGS

A quick and buttery lemon-garlic sauce transforms this fish into something truly spectacular. Pair with tender carrots (one of my favorite veggies to roast because of their natural sweetness), and you won't be disappointed!

1 pound (455 g) carrots, peeled and cut into sticks

4 tablespoons (56 g) ghee, melted, or (60 ml) extra-virgin olive oil, divided

¾ teaspoon salt, divided

4 mahi mahi fillets (see Note) (6 to 8 ounces, or 170 to 225 g, each)

1½ tablespoons (25 ml) fresh lemon juice

1 tablespoon (10 g) minced garlic

1 tablespoon (4 g) chopped fresh parsley

Preheat the oven to 425°F (220°C, or gas mark 7).

Spread the carrots in one half of a 9 x 13-inch (23 x 33 cm) baking dish. Top with 2 tablespoons (28 g) of the ghee and ¼ teaspoon of the salt. Bake for 15 minutes.

Remove from the oven and reduce the temperature to 375°F (190°C, or gas mark 5).

Add the mahi mahi beside the carrots. Top the fish with the remaining 2 tablespoons (28 g) ghee, remaining ½ teaspoon salt, lemon juice, and garlic. Bake until the fish is opaque and flakes easily with a fork, 9 to 10 minutes.

To serve, divide the carrots among plates, along with a piece of fish. Sprinkle the fresh parsley over the mahi mahi.

Note

You can easily swap out the mahi mahi for another fish if you like. Tilapia or flounder would work well!

Barbecue Chicken Thighs with Spicy Broccoli

YIELD: 4 SERVINGS

I love using chicken thighs rather than chicken breasts when possible because they are close to impossible to overcook and stay so juicy! You will appreciate how tender these are. Slather them with a surprisingly easy homemade and sugar-free barbecue sauce for the perfect entree paired with crispy broccoli.

CHICKEN THIGHS & SPICY BROCCOLI

1½ to 1¾ pounds (680 to 795 g) boneless, skinless chicken thighs

3 tablespoons (45 ml) extra-virgin olive oil, divided

½ teaspoon salt, plus more to taste

Black pepper, to taste

12 ounces (340 g) broccoli florets

¼ teaspoon garlic powder

¼ teaspoon crushed red pepper flakes

BARBECUE SAUCE

1 cup (240 g) ketchup

½ cup (120 ml) coconut aminos

2 teaspoons chili powder

1½ teaspoons ground mustard

1 teaspoon apple cider vinegar

1 teaspoon minced garlic

1 teaspoon salt

¼ teaspoon garlic powder

Make the Chicken Thighs with Spicy Broccoli: Preheat the oven to 425°F (220°C, or gas mark 7).

Pat the chicken thighs dry. Rub 1 tablespoon (15 ml) of the oil on the chicken, focusing most of it on the top. Place the chicken on one side of a 12 x 17-inch (30 x 43 cm) sheet pan. Sprinkle with salt and black pepper.

Spread the broccoli in an even layer beside the chicken. Drizzle with the remaining 2 tablespoons (28 ml) oil. Sprinkle with the ½ teaspoon salt, garlic powder, and red pepper flakes.

Bake for 10 minutes.

Meanwhile, make the Barbecue Sauce: In a medium bowl, combine the ketchup, coconut aminos, chili powder, mustard, vinegar, garlic, salt, and garlic powder. Divide between two bowls and set aside.

Remove the chicken and broccoli from the oven and brush the chicken with half of the sauce. Reserve the remaining sauce for later.

Bake for another 10 minutes. To crisp the top of the chicken a bit, broil for 2 to 3 minutes after the baking time finishes.

Remove from the oven. Brush the remaining half of the sauce on top of the chicken. Cover the sheet pan with aluminum foil. Let the chicken rest for 10 minutes so that it's tender and completely cooked through to a minimum internal temperature of 165°F (74°C).

Sheet-Pan Sausage & Veggies

YIELD: 4 SERVINGS

This is the meal I turn to on those busy weeknights when I'm just barely holding on until bedtime. It just doesn't get much easier than this. Chop. Drizzle. Sprinkle. Bake. BOOM. Dinner is served.

PALEO SIMPLE

1 pound (455 g) green beans, trimmed and halved

1 pound (455 g) Brussels sprouts, trimmed and halved

4 fully cooked chicken sausages, sliced ¼-inch (6 mm) thick

3 tablespoons (45 ml) extra-virgin olive oil

Salt and black pepper to taste

1 tablespoon (10 g) minced garlic

Preheat the oven to 425°F (220°C, or gas mark 7).

Spread the green beans, Brussels sprouts, and sausage on a 12 x 17-inch (30 x 43 cm) baking sheet in a single layer.

Drizzle the oil over everything and sprinkle with salt and black pepper. Stir everything together so the oil is evenly distributed and then spread in a single layer.

Bake for 15 minutes.

Remove from the oven and add the garlic. Bake until the vegetables are tender with some crispy edges, another 5 to 10 minutes.

Notes

Any fully cooked sausage will work well here, so feel free to use your favorite brand or go with turkey or beef.

Green beans or Brussels sprouts can be swapped out for another veggie with a similar cooking time. Carrot sticks or diced potatoes (if diced fairly small) would be delicious!

Baked Fish & Root Vegetables

YIELD: 4 SERVINGS

Roasting root vegetables caramelizes the natural sugar in them to bring out their sweetness. Combine that with a flaky white fish, here we are using cod, and you have one incredible meal!

ROOT VEGETABLES

2 cups (244 g) peeled, sliced carrots, ¼-inch (6 mm)-thick slices

2 cups (266 g) diced sweet potatoes, ½-inch (1 cm) cubes

1 red onion, sliced into large chunks

¼ cup (60 ml) extra-virgin olive oil

1 teaspoon salt

½ teaspoon black pepper

FISH

1½ tablespoons (25 ml) fresh lemon juice

1 tablespoon (4 g) finely chopped fresh parsley

1 teaspoon extra-virgin olive oil

¼ teaspoon salt

¼ teaspoon garlic powder

4 cod fillets (6 ounces, or 170 g, each)

Make the Root Vegetables: Preheat the oven to 450°F (230°C, or gas mark 8). Line a 12 x 17-inch (30 x 43 cm) baking sheet with parchment paper.

Spread the carrots, sweet potatoes, and onion on the prepared baking sheet in a single layer.

Drizzle the oil over the veggies and sprinkle with the salt and black pepper. Stir it all together so everything is coated. Spread in a single layer and then bake for 10 minutes.

Meanwhile, make the Fish: Combine the lemon juice, parsley, oil, salt, and garlic powder in a small bowl. Set aside.

Remove the pan from the oven and reduce the temperature to 425°F (220°C, or gas mark 7). Use a spatula to stir the vegetables. Spread in an even layer and create four holes or spaces on the baking sheet for your fish. Add the cod to the pan. Drizzle your lemon juice mixture over the top of the cod.

Bake until the fish is opaque and flakes easily with a fork and the vegetables are tender, 10 to 15 minutes.

Almond-Crusted Chicken Dinner

YIELD: 4 SERVINGS

If you are new to breading chicken with almond flour, you are going to be so pleased with how these chicken cutlets turn out. Perfectly breaded and seasoned chicken with lemony asparagus deserves a place on your menu.

ALMOND-CRUSTED CHICKEN CUTLET

2 tablespoons (28 ml) extra-virgin olive oil

1¼ cups (140 g) finely ground almond flour

¾ teaspoon chili powder

¾ teaspoon garlic powder

¾ teaspoon dried parsley

¾ teaspoon dried basil

¾ teaspoon salt

2 large eggs

2 tablespoons (28 ml) coconut aminos

1 to 1½ pounds (455 to 680 g) chicken breast cutlets, thinly sliced

ASPARAGUS

1 bunch asparagus, trimmed (thick stalk works best)

1 tablespoon (15 ml) extra-virgin olive oil

Juice from ½ lemon

¼ teaspoon salt

Make the Almond-Crusted Chicken Cutlet: Preheat the oven to 450°F (230°C, or gas mark 8). Grease a 12 x 17-inch (30 x 43 cm) baking sheet with the oil.

In a shallow dish, combine the almond flour, chili powder, garlic powder, parsley, basil, and salt. Mix well.

In separate bowl, whisk together the eggs and coconut aminos.

Dredge each chicken cutlet in the egg mixture and let the excess drip off. Then, dredge each cutlet in the breading mixture.

Place each breaded cutlet on one side of the prepared baking sheet, leaving room for the asparagus later. Bake for 12 minutes.

Remove the pan from the oven. Carefully flip each cutlet. Be gentle so the breading doesn't stick to the pan.

Make the Asparagus: Add the asparagus beside the chicken. Drizzle with the oil and lemon juice. Sprinkle with the salt. Bake until the chicken is cooked through to a minimum internal temperature of 165°F (74°C), about 8 minutes more. (If using boneless pork chops, cook to a minimum internal temperature of 145°F [63°C].)

Notes

To bread your chicken, lay a cutlet on top of the breading ingredients and use your fingers to cover the top of the cutlet with breading and press it into the chicken. Breading will stick to the bottom of your cutlet while you do this.

Feel free to swap out the chicken for boneless pork chops.

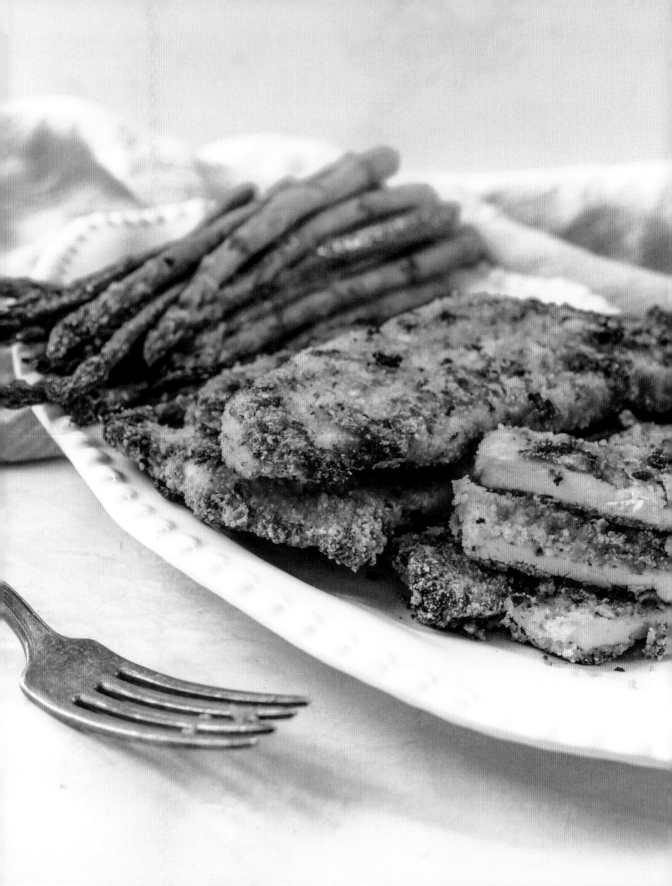

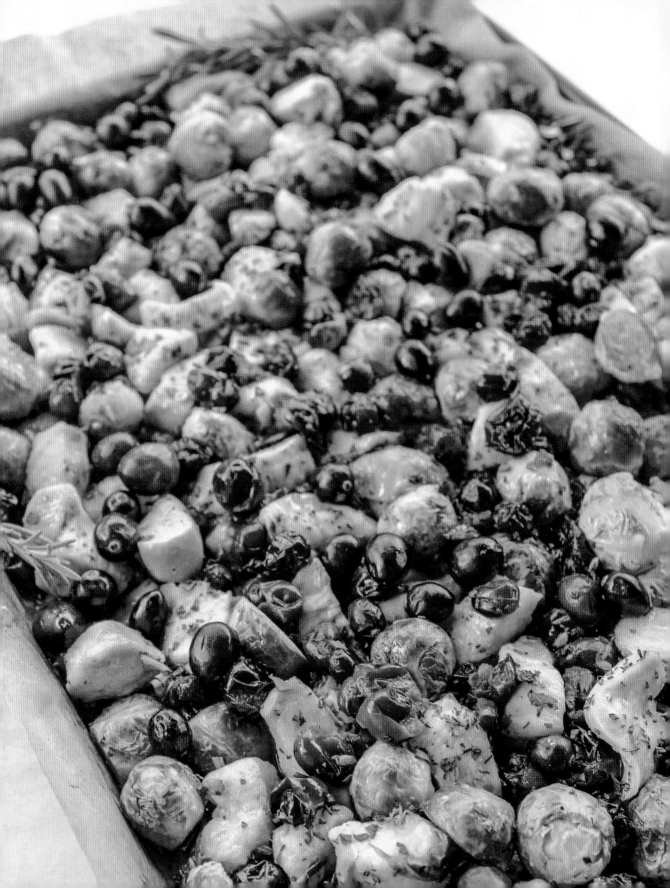

Roasted Cranberry Chicken & Brussels Sprouts

YIELD: 6 TO 8 SERVINGS

Tart fresh cranberries burst as you roast them and add so much flavor to this chicken. I love it paired with crispy roasted Brussels sprouts! Cubed pork tenderloin would also be divine here, so feel free to swap out the chicken, if you want to change things up.

2 pounds (900 g) Brussels sprouts, trimmed and halved (if large)

12 ounces (340 g) fresh cranberries

4 tablespoons (60 ml) extra-virgin olive oil, divided

2 tablespoons (28 ml) pure maple syrup

2 tablespoons (28 ml) coconut aminos

2 pounds (900 g) boneless, skinless chicken breasts, cut into 1-inch (2.5 cm) pieces

1 tablespoon (2 g) finely chopped fresh rosemary

1½ teaspoons salt

Preheat the oven to 425°F (220°C, or gas mark 7). Line a 12 x 17-inch (30 x 43 cm) baking sheet with parchment paper.

Spread the Brussels sprouts and cranberries in an even layer on the prepared baking sheet. Drizzle 2 tablespoons (28 ml) of the oil over everything. Bake for 5 minutes.

Meanwhile, add the remaining 2 tablespoons (28 ml) oil, maple syrup, and coconut aminos to a small bowl. Stir until combined.

Remove the pan from the oven and add the chicken, mixing it in with the Brussels sprouts and cranberries. It's a tight fit, but it will fit. Pour the syrup mixture over everything and sprinkle with the rosemary and salt. Use a spatula to move the Brussels sprouts, cranberries, and chicken around so it's all well coated. Spread in an even layer.

Bake until the chicken is cooked through, completely opaque and juices run clear, about 15 minutes.

Chimichurri Steak Dinner

YIELD: 8 SERVINGS

I personally don't think you can go wrong with steak drizzled in any sauce, but this chimichurri is just extra special. It's tangy and has a little heat. And I would be remiss if I failed to mention how incredible these Brussels sprouts are, my friend. The marinade from the steak makes its way to the veggies as everything cooks, and it is pure magic.

STEAK & BRUSSELS SPROUTS

2 tablespoons (28 ml) coconut aminos

3 tablespoons (45 ml) extra-virgin olive oil, divided

1½ teaspoons salt, divided

½ teaspoon chili powder

½ teaspoon black pepper

2 pounds (900 g) sirloin steak, cut into strips ½-inch (1 cm) thick and 3 to 4 inches (7.5 to 10 cm) long

2 pounds (900 g) Brussels sprouts, trimmed and halved (if large)

CHIMICHURRI SAUCE

½ cup (30 g) tightly packed fresh parsley

3 tablespoons (45 ml) red wine vinegar

2 tablespoons (8 g) chopped fresh oregano

2 tablespoons (20 g) minced garlic

1 teaspoon crushed red pepper flakes

¼ teaspoon salt

¼ cup (60 ml) extra-virgin olive oil

Make the Steak & Brussels Sprouts: Preheat the oven to 425°F (220°C, or gas mark 7).

In a large bowl, combine the coconut aminos, 1 tablespoon (15 ml) of the oil, ¾ teaspoon of the salt, chili powder, and black pepper. Add the steak and toss to coat with the marinade. Set aside.

Spread the Brussels sprouts on one side of a 12 x 17-inch (30 x 43 cm) baking sheet. Drizzle with the remaining 2 tablespoons (28 ml) oil and sprinkle with the remaining ¾ teaspoon salt. Bake for 10 minutes.

Remove the pan from the oven. Add the marinated steak beside the Brussels sprouts. Bake until the steak is cooked how you like it and the Brussels sprouts are tender, 8 to 10 minutes.

Meanwhile, make the Chimichurri Sauce: Add the parsley, vinegar, oregano, garlic, red pepper flakes, and salt to a food processor. Pulse until the herbs are finely chopped. Slowly pour in the oil while pulsing. Scrape down the sides of the food processor if needed.

To serve, divide the Brussels sprouts and steak among plates. Drizzle your Chimichurri Sauce over the steak.

Ghee Chicken with Sweet Sautéed Carrots

YIELD: 4 SERVINGS

How about a simple and easy-to-throw-together dinner? First, we'll sauté our chicken thighs in ghee until they're deliciously browned. Add in some tender, honeyed carrots, and you're all done. The nuttiness of the ghee beautifully complements the sweetness of the carrots for a delicious meal!

1½ pounds (680 g) boneless, skinless chicken thighs

½ teaspoon salt

½ teaspoon garlic powder

3 tablespoons (42 g) ghee, divided

1 pound (455 g) carrots, peeled and sliced ¼-inch (6 mm) thick

1 tablespoon (20 g) raw honey

Pat the chicken thighs dry. Rub the salt and garlic powder into the top of the chicken.

Place 1 tablespoon (14 g) of the ghee in a skillet over medium-high heat. Once hot, add the chicken, seasoned-side down. (You should hear a sizzle.) Flip once you see a beautiful brown on the side of the chicken in the pan, 3 to 4 minutes. Brown the other side, about another 3 minutes. The chicken will not be completely cooked through at this point.

Reduce the heat to medium. Use a spatula to move the chicken to one side of the pan. Add the carrots, 3 tablespoons (45 ml) water, honey, and remaining 2 tablespoons (28 g) ghee. Cover and simmer until the carrots are tender and the chicken is cooked through to a minimum internal temperature of 165°F (74°C), 5 to 7 minutes. Taste and add more salt, if desired.

Note

Feel free to swap out the chicken thighs for chicken breasts. Breasts generally require less overall cooking time, depending on the thickness.

Orange Chicken Cauliflower Rice Bowls

YIELD: 4 SERVINGS

Cauliflower rice bowls are such a fun way to load up on veggies without feeling like you are loading up on veggies! I enjoy playing around with different flavor combinations, and this one features roasted veggies and chicken in a sticky orange sauce. Don't skip the zest!

CHICKEN & VEGGIES

12 ounces (340 g) fresh green beans, trimmed and halved

3 tablespoons (45 ml) extra-virgin olive oil, divided

2 cups (8 ounces, or 225 g) cauliflower rice

1 yellow or orange bell pepper, sliced into strips

1½ pounds (680 g) boneless, skinless chicken breasts, cut into 1-inch (2.5 cm) pieces

½ teaspoon salt

½ teaspoon garlic powder

ORANGE SAUCE

3 tablespoons (45 ml) fresh orange juice

2½ tablespoons (50 g) raw honey

1 tablespoon (15 ml) coconut aminos

1 tablespoon (6 g) orange zest

1 tablespoon (9 g) arrowroot flour

1 tablespoon (15 ml) cold water

Make the Chicken & Veggies: Preheat the oven to 400°F (200°C, or gas mark 6).

Add the green beans to a 12 x 17-inch (30 x 43 cm) baking sheet in a single layer. Drizzle 1 tablespoon (15 ml) of the oil on top. Bake for 5 minutes.

Meanwhile, prepare your Orange Sauce: Combine the orange juice, honey, coconut aminos, and orange zest in a small bowl. In a small jar, shake together the arrowroot flour and water to create a slurry. Stir the slurry into the sauce. Set aside.

Remove the green beans from the oven. Use a spatula to carefully move them to one side of the pan. Spread the cauliflower rice beside it, then the bell peppers, and then the chicken.

Drizzle the remaining 2 tablespoons (28 ml) oil over the bell peppers and cauliflower rice. Sprinkle the salt over everything on the baking sheet. Add the garlic powder to the chicken and green beans.

Pour the Orange Sauce over the chicken only. Use a spatula to move the chicken around in the sauce so the chicken is coated.

Bake for 10 minutes. The sauce will get bubbly as it heats up in the oven. That's great!

Remove from the oven and separate the chicken if it's sticking together. Use a spatula to push the sauce to the chicken if it's running into the vegetables. Return to the oven and bake until the chicken is cooked through, completely opaque and juices run clear, about 5 additional minutes.

Remove from the oven. Layer your cauliflower rice, green beans, bell pepper, and chicken in bowls. Top with any sauce remaining in the pan.

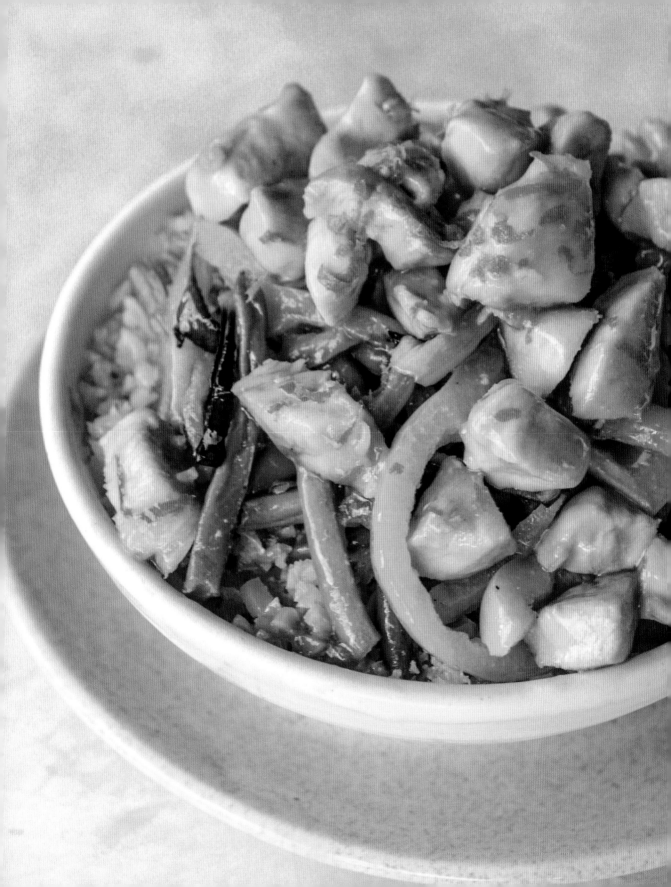

Easy Italian Sausage & Peppers

YIELD: 4 SERVINGS

This Italian-inspired meal includes the hard-to-beat flavor combo of sausage, onion, and bell peppers. Add in fresh basil and throw it over roasted cauliflower rice for a seriously spectacular dinner that will earn rave reviews in your home.

12 ounces (340 g) fully cooked chicken sausages, sliced ¼-inch (6 mm) thick

1 red bell pepper, sliced into thin strips

1 yellow or orange bell pepper, sliced into thin strips

1 white or yellow onion, sliced into thin strips

4 tablespoons (60 ml) extra-virgin olive oil, divided

½ teaspoon garlic powder

½ teaspoon dried oregano

½ teaspoon dried basil

¾ teaspoon salt, divided

½ teaspoon black pepper

3 cups (12 ounces, or 340 g) cauliflower rice

5 or 6 large basil leaves, chopped

Preheat the oven to 425°F (220°C, or gas mark 7).

Spread the chicken sausage, bell peppers, and onion on a 12 x 17-inch (30 x 43 cm) baking sheet. Drizzle with 3 tablespoons (45 ml) of the oil, garlic powder, oregano, dried basil, ½ teaspoon of the salt, and black pepper. Use a spoon or spatula to stir so everything is evenly coated and then gently push the mixture to one side so you have enough room for your cauliflower rice.

Spread the cauliflower rice on the other side. Add the remaining 1 table-spoon (15 ml) oil and remaining ¼ teaspoon salt on top of the cauliflower.

Bake until the peppers and onions are tender, about 20 minutes.

Garnish with the fresh basil after baking. To serve, layer the cauliflower rice in bowls and top with the sausage, bell peppers, and onion.

Pistachio-Herb Crusted Salmon with Asparagus

YIELD: 4 SERVINGS

Just wait until you try the crust on this salmon! Made from pistachios, basil, and lemon juice, it's thick, so it really clings to the top of your gorgeous fish as it roasts. I highly recommend this for even the pickiest seafood eater!

PISTACHIO-HERB CRUSTED SALMON

4 wild-caught salmon fillets (6 ounces, or 170 g, each)

½ cup (12 g) fresh basil

⅓ cup (41 g) shelled pistachios

2 tablespoons (28 ml) extra-virgin olive oil

2 tablespoons (28 ml) fresh lemon juice

½ teaspoon salt

½ teaspoon black pepper

ASPARAGUS

1 bunch fresh asparagus, trimmed

1 tablespoon (15 ml) extra-virgin olive oil

Salt, to taste

Make the Pistachio-Herb Crusted Salmon: Preheat the oven to 425°F (220°C, or gas mark 7).

Place the salmon, skin-side down, on a nonstick baking sheet or on a 12 x 17-inch (30 x 43 cm) baking sheet lined with parchment paper.

To a food processor or high-powered blender, add the basil, pistachios, oil, lemon juice, salt, and black pepper. Blend until you don't have any large chunks of pistachio.

Spread the mixture over the top of each salmon fillet. You'll want to use every single bit. (It's really good!)

Bake for 5 minutes. Remove from the oven.

Make the Asparagus: Add the asparagus to the baking sheet beside your salmon. Drizzle with the oil and sprinkle with salt.

Bake until the salmon is cooked through, opaque and flakes easily with a fork, and the asparagus is slightly wilted but still crunchy, an additional 8 to 10 minutes.

Mediterranean Fish Dinner

YIELD: 4 SERVINGS

For this recipe, I bake cod with classic Mediterranean ingredients like tomatoes, olives, and capers. Lemon brightens up this dish, and it's all a total feast for the eyes as well as the stomach!

2½ tablespoons (40 ml) extra-virgin olive oil

2 medium zucchini, halved and sliced into half-moons (about 4 cups, or 480 g)

4 cod fillets (6 ounces, or 170 g, each)

1 cup (180 g) grape tomatoes

¾ cup (75 g) pitted kalamata olives

2 tablespoons (18 g) capers

1 teaspoon minced garlic

1 teaspoon salt

½ teaspoon black pepper

1 lemon, thinly sliced

2 tablespoons (8 g) chopped fresh parsley

Preheat the oven to 425°F (220°C, or gas mark 7). Coat the bottom of a 9 x 13-inch (23 x 33 cm) baking dish with the oil.

Spread the zucchini across the bottom of the baking dish. Lay the cod on top so the fillets do not touch.

Place the tomatoes, olives, capers, and garlic on top of the zucchini in the spaces between the cod. Sprinkle the salt and black pepper over everything.

Place the lemon slices on top of the cod.

Bake until the fish is opaque and flakes easily with a fork and the zucchini is tender, 15 to 20 minutes. Garnish with the parsley before serving.

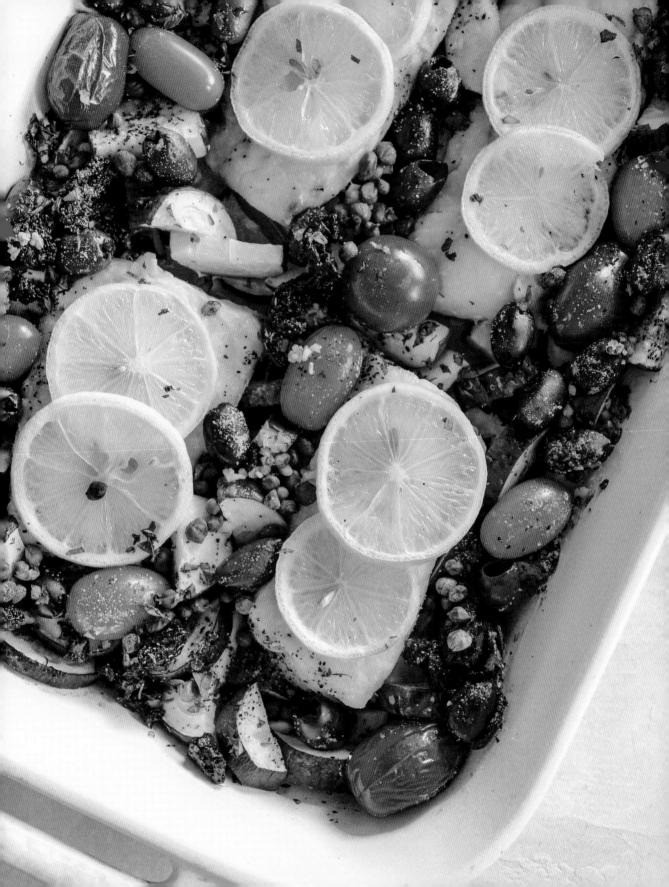

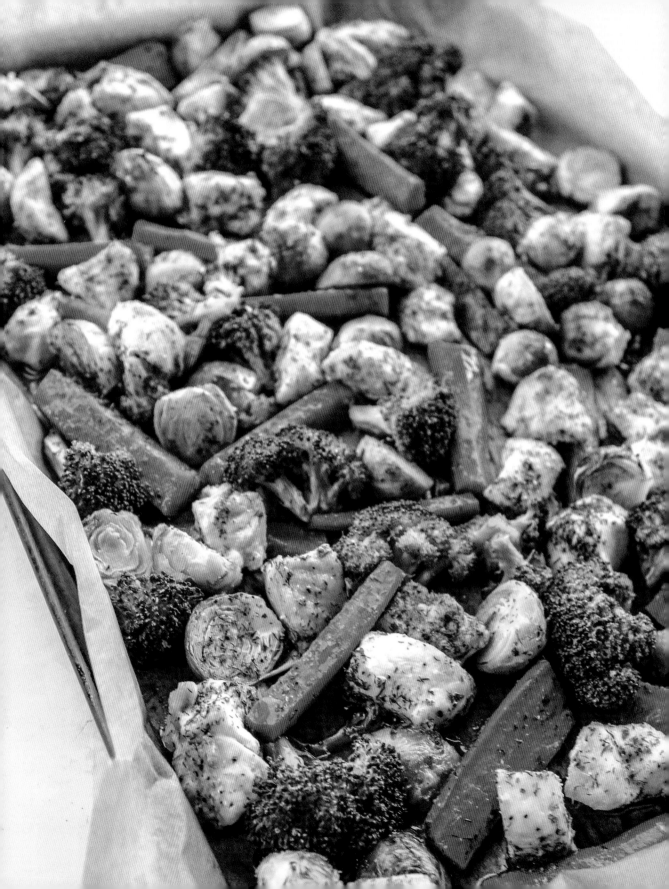

Harvest Ranch Chicken Dinner

YIELD: 4 TO 6 SERVINGS

Ranch seasoning is so easy to make at home and packs so much flavor. In this recipe, we roast chicken, broccoli, carrots, and Brussels sprouts (lots of good veggies!) with this delectable seasoning. Everything gets coated, and the veggies come out perfectly tender with crispy edges. Just how I like them!

CHICKEN & VEGGIES

4 cups (284 g) broccoli florets

2 large carrots, peeled and cut into sticks (about 2 cups, or 244 g)

2 cups (176 g) Brussels sprouts, trimmed and halved

4 tablespoons (60 ml) extra-virgin olive oil, divided

1½ pounds (680 g) boneless, skinless chicken breasts, cut into 1-inch (2.5 cm) pieces

RANCH SEASONING

1 teaspoon dried dill

1 teaspoon dried parsley

1 teaspoon garlic powder

1 teaspoon salt

½ teaspoon onion powder

½ teaspoon black pepper

Make the Chicken & Veggies: Preheat the oven to 425°F (220°C, or gas mark 7). Line a 12 x 17-inch (30 x 43 cm) baking sheet with parchment paper.

Spread the broccoli, carrots, and Brussels sprouts in an even layer on the prepared baking sheet.

Drizzle 2 tablespoons (28 ml) of the oil over the veggies and bake for 5 minutes.

Meanwhile, make the Ranch Seasoning: In a small bowl, combine the dill, parsley, garlic powder, salt, onion powder, and black pepper.

Remove the pan from the oven and add the chicken. Drizzle the remaining 2 tablespoons (28 ml) oil over everything. Add all the Ranch Seasoning. Use a spatula to move the veggies and chicken around so that it's all well coated in oil and seasoning. Spread in a single layer.

Bake until the chicken is cooked through, completely opaque and juices run clear, and the vegetables are tender yet a little crispy, about 15 minutes.

Note

Feel free to swap out the chicken for boneless pork chops, cut into 1-inch (2.5 cm) pieces.

Fiesta Pineapple Chicken

YIELD: 4 SERVINGS

This easy stir-fry of chicken, pineapple, and vegetables is the perfect combination of sweet and savory. It's also so pretty, if I do say so myself!

2 tablespoons (28 ml) extra-virgin olive oil or avocado oil

1 pound (455 g) boneless, skinless chicken breasts, cut into 1-inch (2.5 cm) pieces

1 red bell pepper, cut into 1-inch (2.5 cm) pieces

½ white or yellow onion, cut into 1-inch (2.5 cm) pieces

12 ounces (340 g) green beans, trimmed and halved

¾ teaspoon salt

½ teaspoon black pepper

½ teaspoon ground ginger

1 can (14 ounces, or 390 g) pineapple chunks, drained, or 1½ cups (250 g) fresh

½ cup (120 ml) chicken stock

¼ cup (60 ml) coconut aminos

1½ teaspoons minced garlic

¼ teaspoon crushed red pepper flakes

1 tablespoon (9 g) arrowroot flour

1 tablespoon (15 ml) cold water

Add the oil to the skillet over medium-high heat. Once hot, add the chicken. Sauté, flipping occasionally to brown all sides of the chicken, about 3 to 5 minutes, using a spatula to separate the pieces when they get stuck together. Remove the chicken from the skillet and set aside.

Add the bell pepper, onion, and green beans to the skillet. Sauté, stirring occasionally, until the onion is tender and the bell pepper and green beans have some browning, about 5 minutes.

Add the chicken back to your skillet along with the salt, black pepper, and ginger. Stir in the pineapple chunks.

Stir in the stock, coconut aminos, garlic, and red pepper flakes. Simmer for 2 to 3 minutes until the chicken is cooked through, completely opaque and juices run clear, and everything is warmed through.

Turn off the stove. To thicken the sauce, combine the arrowroot flour and water in a small jar. Shake vigorously and pour the slurry into the skillet and stir. The sauce will begin to thicken immediately.

Taste and add more salt and black pepper, if desired.

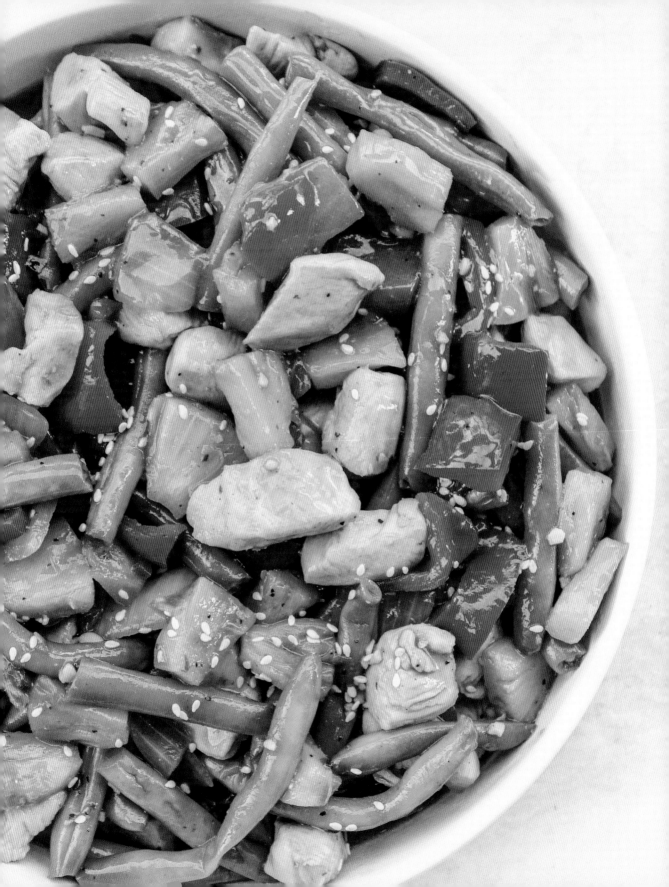

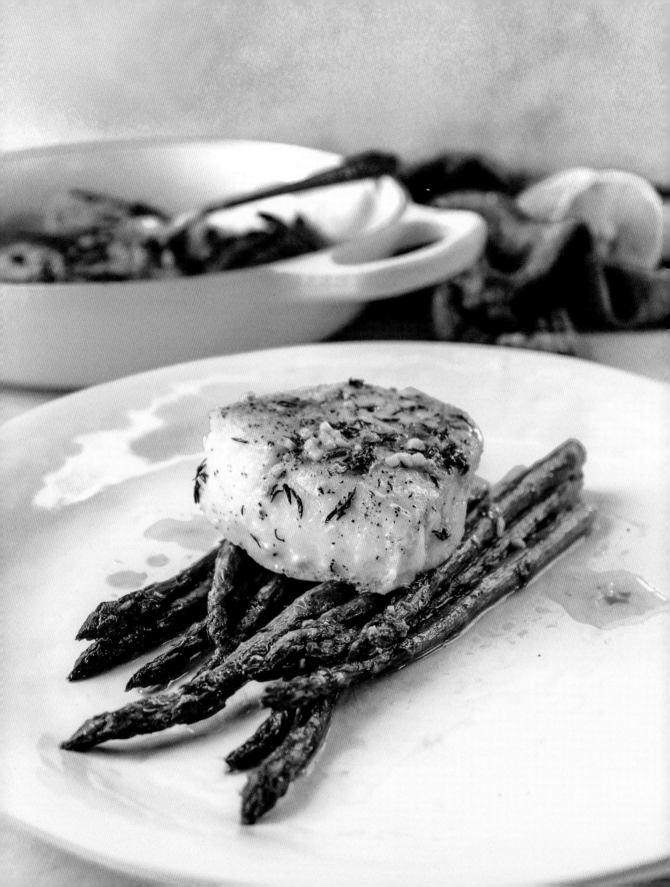

Garlic-Lemon Halibut with Sautéed Asparagus

YIELD: 4 SERVINGS

Halibut has a mild flavor that pleases pretty much everybody. (Even those who protest that they don't really enjoy seafood.) My favorite way to dress it up is with a lovely sauce of ghee, lemon juice, garlic, and thyme. It's just perfect with asparagus!

HALIBUT & ASPARAGUS

4 halibut fillets (6 ounces, or 170 g, each)

Salt and black pepper

2 tablespoons (28 ml) extra-virgin olive oil

1 bunch asparagus, trimmed

GARLIC-LEMON SAUCE

¼ cup (56 g) ghee, melted

2 tablespoons (28 ml) fresh lemon juice

1 tablespoon (2 g) chopped fresh thyme

1 teaspoon minced garlic

Make the Halibut & Asparagus: Generously sprinkle the top and bottom of the halibut with salt and black pepper.

Add the oil to a large skillet over medium-high heat. Once hot, carefully add each fillet with the presentation-side down. Place the asparagus beside the fish and sprinkle with salt. We want a beautiful golden color on the side of the halibut that's touching the bottom of the pan, so don't flip it until you've achieved that color, 4 to 5 minutes.

Meanwhile, make the Garlic-Lemon Sauce: Stir together the ghee, lemon juice, thyme, and garlic in a small bowl.

Carefully flip your halibut and use your spatula or tongs to move the asparagus around so all the stalks get a turn at the bottom of the pan.

Reduce the heat to medium-low or low. Pour your ghee mixture over the halibut and asparagus. Cover and let the halibut cook through until it is opaque and flakes easily with a fork, 3 to 4 minutes.

To serve, divide the asparagus among plates and top with the halibut. Drizzle a bit of the sauce from the pan over the fish.

Crispy Chicken Thighs with Greens

YIELD: 4 SERVINGS

Get your greens in this simple dish of lightly spiced chicken thighs and garlicky spinach. You can swap out the spinach for any other fast-cooking green veggie and make this seem like a new dish every time you make it!

CHICKEN THIGHS

½ teaspoon salt

½ teaspoon chili powder

½ teaspoon garlic powder

½ teaspoon black pepper

¼ teaspoon curry powder

¼ teaspoon paprika

1½ pounds (680 g) boneless, skinless chicken thighs

1½ tablespoons (21 g) ghee (see Notes)

SPINACH

½ to 1½ teaspoons extra-virgin olive oil

15 ounces (425 g) fresh baby spinach (see Notes)

1½ teaspoons minced garlic

½ teaspoon salt

Make the Chicken Thighs: In a small bowl, stir together the salt, chili powder, garlic powder, black pepper, curry powder, and paprika.

Pat the chicken thighs dry. Rub the spice mixture into the top of the chicken.

Place the ghee in a skillet over medium-high heat. Once hot, add the chicken, seasoned-side down. (You should hear a sizzle.) Flip once you see a beautiful brown on the side of the chicken in the pan, 5 minutes. Brown the other side, another 6 to 7 minutes. Remove the chicken from the pan and set aside.

Make the Spinach: Reduce the heat to medium. Assess how much fat remains in the skillet. You may find that you don't need to add any oil, or you may only need a little. Add the oil (if needed), spinach, garlic, and salt. Stir until all the spinach fits. Place the chicken thighs on top of the spinach. Cover and simmer until the chicken is cooked through to a minimum internal temperature of 165°F (74°C) and the spinach is wilted, 2 to 4 minutes.

Notes

Use another cooking fat in place of ghee if you like. I personally really enjoy the rich flavor of ghee for sautéing chicken.

Interested in using something other than spinach? Mustard greens cook quickly, so they're a great swap; tear or chop the greens into large pieces before sautéing. If you'd like to use kale, remove the thickest part of the stems first and then give the leaves a rough chop; cook kale for 6 to 8 minutes. Broccoli cooks fast, too; just move those thighs to the side of your skillet, add the broccoli, and cover and cook until it's how you like it!

Easy Roast Chicken

YIELD: 4–6 SERVINGS

Here's a simple recipe that results in a juicy roast with crispy skin. It's great served fresh, and then you can use the leftover meat for other meals.

4- to 5-pound (1.8–2.3 kg) whole chicken

2 tablespoons (30 ml) melted ghee

1 tablespoon (15 ml) garlic-infused olive oil

Zest and juice of 1 lemon

1 teaspoon salt

¼ teaspoon ground black pepper

Preheat the oven to 375°F (190°C or gas mark 5). Place the chicken in a roasting pan or on a rimmed baking sheet. Remove the giblets from inside the chicken and discard or save for another use.

Stir together the ghee, olive oil, lemon zest, and lemon juice in a small bowl. Drizzle over the chicken, making sure it's coated well.

Sprinkle with the salt and pepper and bake for 70–80 minutes, or until the meat reaches 165°F (74°C) on a meat thermometer at the thickest part.

Let the chicken rest for 10 minutes. Slice the chicken, transfer to a platter, and serve.

Store leftovers, covered, in the refrigerator for up to 6 days.

Lemon Shrimp Stir-Fry

YIELD: 4 SERVINGS

Dinner in 20 minutes? This is the stir-fry for you! Shrimp, bell pepper, broccoli, and snow peas simmer in a flavorful lemon sauce. It's so delicious and easy!

LEMON SAUCE

⅔ cup (160 ml) vegetable stock

¼ cup (60 ml) fresh lemon juice

1½ teaspoons minced garlic

1½ teaspoons chopped fresh rosemary

1 teaspoon coconut aminos

¼ teaspoon rice vinegar

¼ teaspoon crushed red pepper flakes

¼ teaspoon salt

¼ teaspoon black pepper

SHRIMP STIR-FRY

1 pound (455 g) peeled and deveined shrimp (16 to 20 count)

Salt and black pepper

2 tablespoons (28 ml) extra-virgin olive oil

1 red bell pepper, sliced into strips

1 yellow or orange bell pepper, sliced into strips

12 ounces (340 g) broccoli florets

8 ounces (225 g) snow peas or fresh green beans (see Note)

Lemon zest, for garnish (optional)

Fresh chopped parsley, for garnish (optional)

Make the Lemon Sauce: Whisk together the stock, lemon juice, garlic, rosemary, coconut aminos, vinegar, red pepper flakes, salt, and black pepper in a small bowl. Set aside.

Make the Shrimp Stir-Fry: Sprinkle the shrimp with salt and black pepper.

Add the oil to a large skillet over medium-high heat. When hot, add the bell peppers and broccoli. Sauté, stirring frequently, until the peppers have started to soften and you're getting some browning, 4 to 5 minutes.

Pour the Lemon Sauce into the skillet and add the shrimp. Carefully stir so everything is well combined. Place the snow peas on top. (Do not stir or the peas will turn to mush.) Cover and simmer until the shrimp is curled and no longer pink, 2 to 3 minutes.

Garnish with lemon zest and parsley before serving, if desired.

Note

If using green beans instead of snow peas, add them to the skillet with the bell peppers and broccoli. They'll take longer to cook than the snow peas, which are very thin and require minimal cooking time.

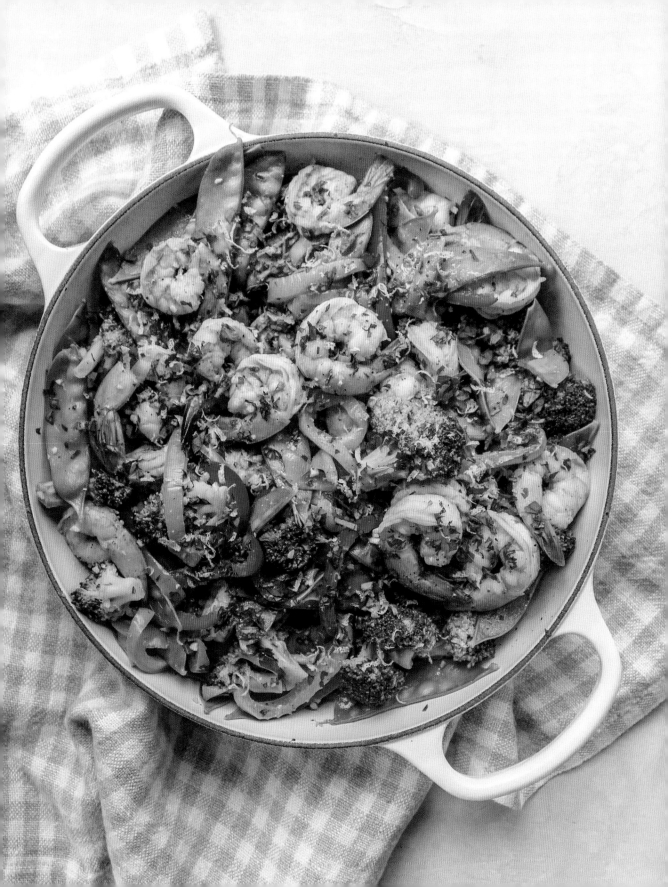

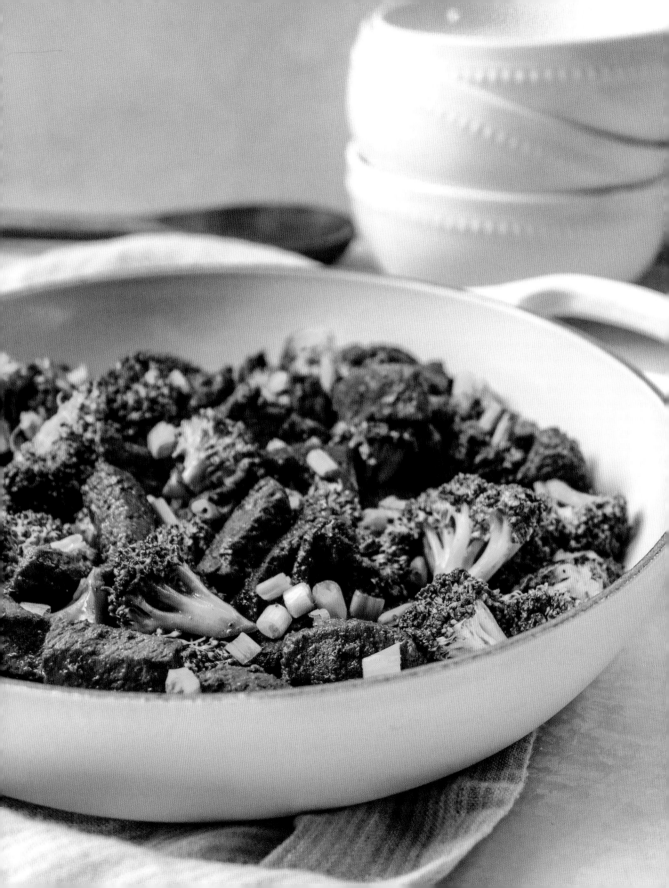

Beef & Broccoli

YIELD: 4 SERVINGS

This beef and broccoli is faster than takeout and so much healthier too! This dish is packed with tender strips of sirloin in an easy marinade and crunchy broccoli florets. The marinade works its magic in as little as 15 minutes, but you can get the meat going in the morning, if you prefer, and then you'll be ready to cook at dinnertime. The whole family will adore this one! It's hearty enough as is, but enjoy it over steamed cauliflower rice for an even more satisfying meal.

MARINADE & BEEF

⅓ cup (80 ml) coconut aminos

1 teaspoon minced garlic

1 teaspoon ground ginger

½ teaspoon salt

½ teaspoon black pepper

½ teaspoon garlic powder

½ teaspoon onion powder

1 pound (455 g) sirloin or flank steak, cut into thin strips

2 tablespoons (28 ml) extra-virgin olive oil

BROCCOLI

1 pound (455 g) broccoli florets

Salt and black pepper

1 scallion, sliced, for garnish (optional)

1½ teaspoons sesame seeds, for garnish (optional)

Coconut aminos, for drizzling (optional)

Make the Marinade & Beef: In a resealable plastic bag or bowl, combine the coconut aminos, garlic, ginger, salt, black pepper, garlic powder, and onion powder. Add the steak, seal the bag, and toss to coat. Refrigerate for a minimum of 15 minutes and up to 12 hours before cooking.

Add the oil to a skillet over medium-high heat. Once hot, add the steak in a single layer. (Reserve any marinade that hasn't been absorbed.) Sauté the steak so that all the sides get a bit of crispy browning, about 5 minutes. The beef doesn't need to be completely cooked through before moving to the next step.

Make the Broccoli: Reduce the heat to medium. Add the broccoli, any leftover marinade, ½ cup (120 ml) water, salt, and black pepper. Stir. Cover and let the broccoli steam until it's how you like it, usually 2 to 3 minutes to keep it bright with a little crispiness.

Taste and add extra salt or black pepper, if necessary. Top with scallion, sesame seeds, and/or an extra drizzle of coconut aminos before serving, if desired.

Maple Salmon with Sweet Potatoes

You will not believe what the maple syrup does to the salmon and sweet potatoes in this impressive meal. I swear these are the sweetest, most tender potatoes I've ever had. I can't wait for you to try this showstopper of a dish!

SWEET POTATOES

2 tablespoons (28 g) coconut oil

2 medium sweet potatoes, diced into ¼-inch (6 mm) cubes

½ teaspoon ground cinnamon

⅛ teaspoon salt, plus more to taste

SALMON

4 wild-caught salmon fillets (6 ounces, or 170 g, each)

Black pepper, to taste

1 tablespoon (14 g) ghee

MAPLE SAUCE

¼ cup (60 ml) pure maple syrup

3 tablespoons (45 ml) coconut aminos

2 teaspoons ghee, melted

1 teaspoon minced garlic

Make the Sweet Potatoes: Add the oil to a skillet over medium-high heat. Once hot, add the sweet potatoes, cinnamon, and ⅛ teaspoon of salt. Stir frequently as you sauté for 4 to 5 minutes. Then, cover and cook until softened, another 4 to 5 minutes.

Meanwhile, make the Salmon: Pat the salmon dry. (This will help the skin crisp up as it cooks and will reduce the likelihood of it sticking to the pan.) Sprinkle with salt and black pepper.

Use a spatula to carefully move the sweet potatoes to one side of the skillet. Add the ghee to the empty side. Place the salmon in the ghee, skin-side up. Cook until golden brown on the side pressed into the pan, about 4 minutes.

While the salmon is cooking, make the Maple Sauce: Stir together the maple syrup, coconut aminos, melted ghee, and garlic in a small bowl.

Gently flip the salmon. Pour your Maple Sauce over everything. Cook until the fish is firm to the touch, opaque, and flakes easily with a fork, about 3 minutes.

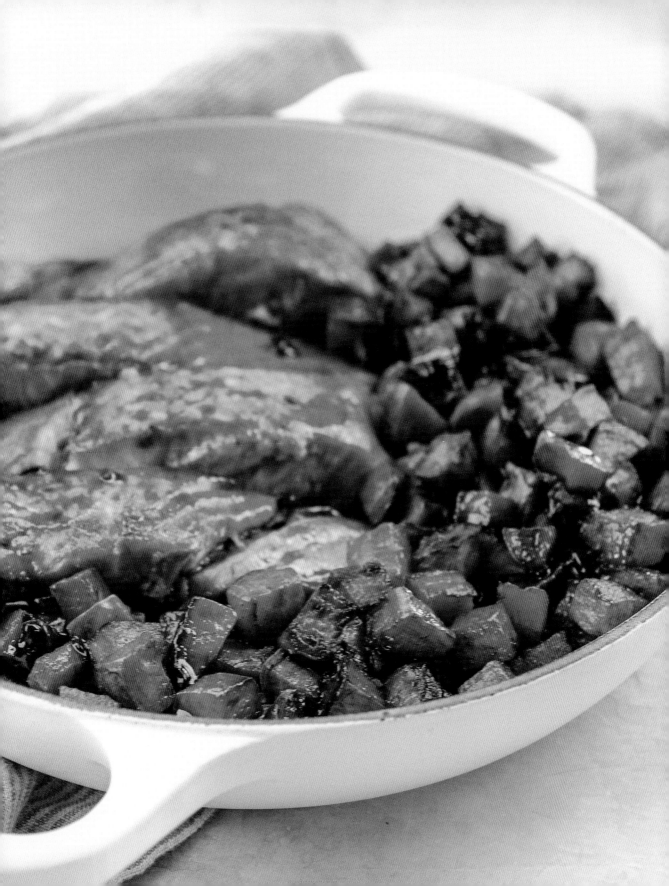

Salsa Chicken & Mexican Cauliflower Rice

YIELD: 2 TO 4 SERVINGS

Lighten up your dinner with this sautéed chicken topped with homemade pico de gallo. Serve it on a bed of Mexican cauliflower rice, and your family will thank you!

CHICKEN

2 boneless, skinless chicken breasts (½ pound, or 225 g, each)

1 teaspoon dried oregano

½ teaspoon salt

½ teaspoon onion powder

½ teaspoon garlic powder

2 tablespoons (28 ml) extra-virgin olive oil

PICO DE GALLO

1 medium tomato, diced into ½-inch (1 cm) or smaller pieces

½ large onion, diced into ½-inch (1 cm) or smaller pieces

¼ to ½ small jalapeño, seeded and diced (optional)

Handful of cilantro, chopped

Lime juice, to taste

Salt, to taste

MEXICAN CAULI-FLOWER RICE

¼ cup (38 g) diced red bell pepper, ½-inch (1 cm) dice

¼ cup (38 g) diced green bell pepper, ½-inch (1 cm) dice

¼ white or yellow onion, diced into ½-inch (1 cm) pieces

1 teaspoon minced garlic

3 cups (12 ounces, or 340 g) fresh or frozen cauliflower rice

2 teaspoons fresh lime juice

½ teaspoon salt

¼ teaspoon chili powder

Make the Chicken: Slice the chicken horizontally to create four thin cutlets. Mix the oregano, salt, onion powder, and garlic powder in a small bowl and press the mixture into the top of the chicken.

Add the oil to a skillet over medium-high heat. Place the chicken, seasoned-side down, in the hot pan. (You should hear a sizzle!) Cook until browned, 3 to 4 minutes. Flip and brown the other side, another 3 minutes. Remove the chicken from the pan and set aside. The chicken does not need to be completely cooked through.

Meanwhile, assemble the Pico de Gallo: In a bowl, stir together the tomato, onion, jalapeño (if using), and cilantro. Add the lime juice and salt a little at a time until you get it how you like it. Set aside.

Make the Mexican Cauliflower Rice: To the skillet, add the bell peppers, onion, and garlic and return to medium-high heat. Scrape up the browned chicken bits remaining in the pan. You should have enough fat left in the pan to sauté with, but if you need more, add an extra tablespoon (15 ml) oil. Sauté until the peppers and onion start to get tender, 2 to 3 minutes.

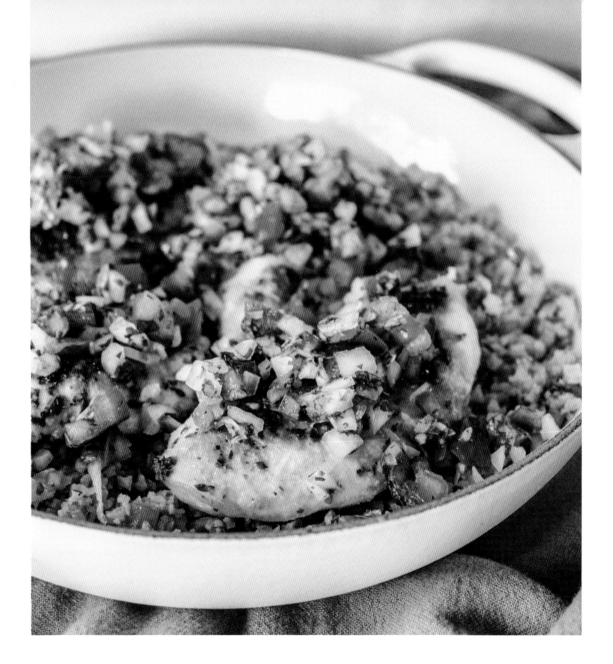

Stir in the cauliflower rice. Add the lime juice, salt, chili powder, and 3 tablespoons (45 ml) water. Place the chicken on top of everything. Reduce the heat to medium, cover, and cook until your cauliflower is tender and your chicken is cooked through, completely opaque and juices run clear, about 5 minutes.

Top the chicken with your homemade Pico de Gallo before serving.

Garlic Crushed Red Pepper Chicken Stir-Fry

YIELD: 4 SERVINGS

You just cannot go wrong with chicken and green beans. This stir-fry has some heat thanks to the crushed red pepper flakes, too. Feel free to swap out the chicken for boneless pork chops if that's what you have on hand.

1 tablespoon (15 ml) extra-virgin olive oil or avocado oil

2 pounds (900 g) boneless, skinless chicken breasts, cut into 1-inch (2.5 cm) pieces

1 teaspoon dried basil

½ teaspoon salt

½ teaspoon black pepper

3 tablespoons (45 ml) coconut aminos

1 tablespoon (15 g) ghee

1½ teaspoons minced garlic

½ teaspoon ground ginger

½ teaspoon crushed red pepper flakes (see Note)

1 pound (455 g) fresh green beans, trimmed and cut into halves or thirds

Sesame seeds, for garnish

Add the oil to a large skillet over medium-high heat. Once hot, add the chicken. Sprinkle the basil, salt, and black pepper on top and stir. Brown on all sides, 3 to 4 minutes. The chicken doesn't need to be completely cooked through at this point.

When the chicken is browned, stir in the coconut aminos, ghee, garlic, ginger, and red pepper flakes. Add the green beans and stir again.

Lower the heat to medium to medium-low. Cover and simmer for 10 minutes, stirring frequently to scrape up the browned bits from the bottom of the pan. (Those are yummy!) The chicken should be cooked through, completely opaque and juices run clear, and the green beans should be softened but not totally wilted.

Sprinkle with the sesame seeds before serving.

Note

If you want to limit the spiciness in this dish, start with ¼ teaspoon red pepper flakes instead of the full ½ teaspoon this recipe calls for.

Skillet Chicken with Summer Vegetables

YIELD: 2 TO 4 SERVINGS

We always have way more squash and zucchini than I know what to do with by the end of summer. Our garden gives us an abundance, and it can get a bit out of hand! This skillet chicken is a delicious way to enjoy our favorite summer veggies. It's an easy dish made of fresh ingredients.

2 boneless, skinless chicken breasts (½ pound, or 225 g each)

2 teaspoons dried basil

1 teaspoon garlic powder, divided

1 teaspoon salt, divided

½ teaspoon onion powder

3 tablespoons (45 ml) extra-virgin olive oil or avocado oil, divided

2 yellow squash, halved and sliced into half-moons

2 medium zucchini, halved and sliced into half-moons

½ white or yellow onion, diced into ½-inch (1 cm) pieces

1 tablespoon (4 g) chopped fresh parsley

Slice the chicken horizontally to create four thin cutlets. Season all sides with the basil, ½ teaspoon of the garlic powder, ½ teaspoon of the salt, and onion powder.

Add 1 tablespoon (15 ml) of the oil to a skillet over medium-high heat. Place the cutlets in the hot pan. (You should hear a little sizzle.) Cook until browned, 3 to 4 minutes. Flip and brown the other side, another 3 to 4 minutes.

Carefully move the chicken to one side of the skillet and reduce the heat to medium. Add the remaining 2 tablespoons (28 ml) oil, squash, zucchini, and onion. Sprinkle with the remaining ½ teaspoon salt and remaining ½ teaspoon garlic powder. Cover and simmer, stirring the veggies occasionally, until the vegetables are tender and the chicken is cooked through to a minimum internal temperature of 165°F (74°C), 5 to 7 minutes. (If using pork cutlets, cook to a minimum internal temperature of 145°F [63°C].)

Garnish with the parsley before serving. Taste and add salt, if desired.

Note

Swap out the chicken for thin-sliced pork cutlets, if you like.

Bourbon Chicken

YIELD: 4 TO 6 SERVINGS

This used to be my favorite dish to buy from the mall food court. This remake, named after the famed street in New Orleans, has much less sugar, but it still has all the flavor! It's delicious served with zucchini noodles or cauliflower rice.

1 tablespoon (15 ml) garlic-infused olive oil

2 pounds (907 g) boneless skinless chicken breasts, cut into 1-inch (3 cm) pieces

½ teaspoon salt

¼ teaspoon ground black pepper

¼ cup (60 ml) apple juice

2 tablespoons (30 ml) ketchup, homemade or paleo store-bought (such as Primal Kitchen)

⅓ cup (80 ml) coconut aminos

½ cup (120 ml) water

¼ teaspoon ground ginger

1 tablespoon (10 g) arrowroot powder/starch

Heat the olive oil in a large skillet over medium heat. Add the chicken, salt, and pepper. Cook, stirring regularly, for 5 minutes. The chicken will not be fully cooked at this point. Transfer to a plate.

Add the apple juice, ketchup, coconut aminos, water, and ginger. Cook for 10 minutes, or until slightly reduced. Add the arrowroot powder, whisk to combine, and stir with a spoon for about 2 minutes, or until the sauce thickens. Add the chicken back in and cook for 10 minutes, or until the chicken is cooked through. Serve warm.

Store leftovers, covered, in the refrigerator for up to 6 days.

PALEO SIMPLE

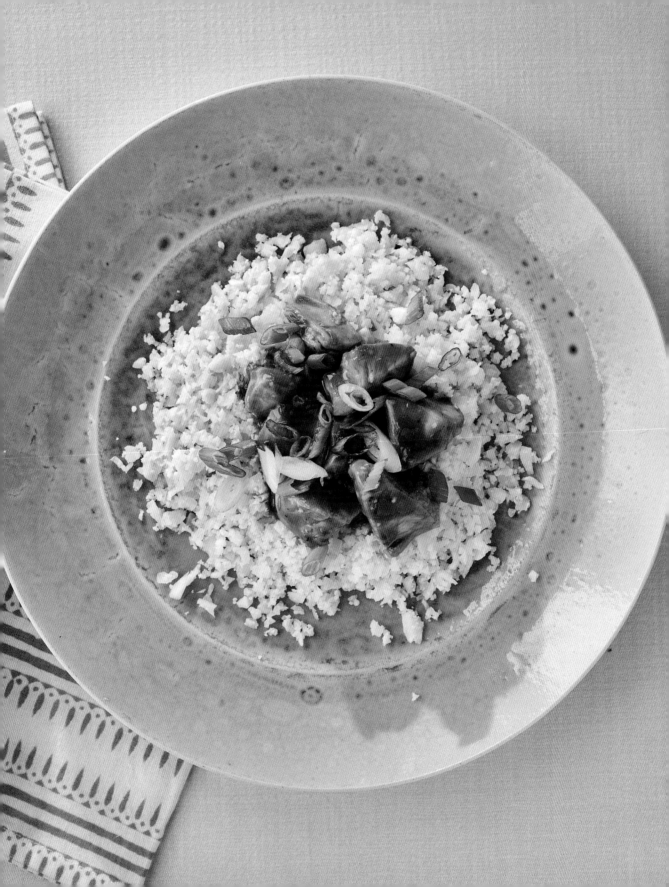

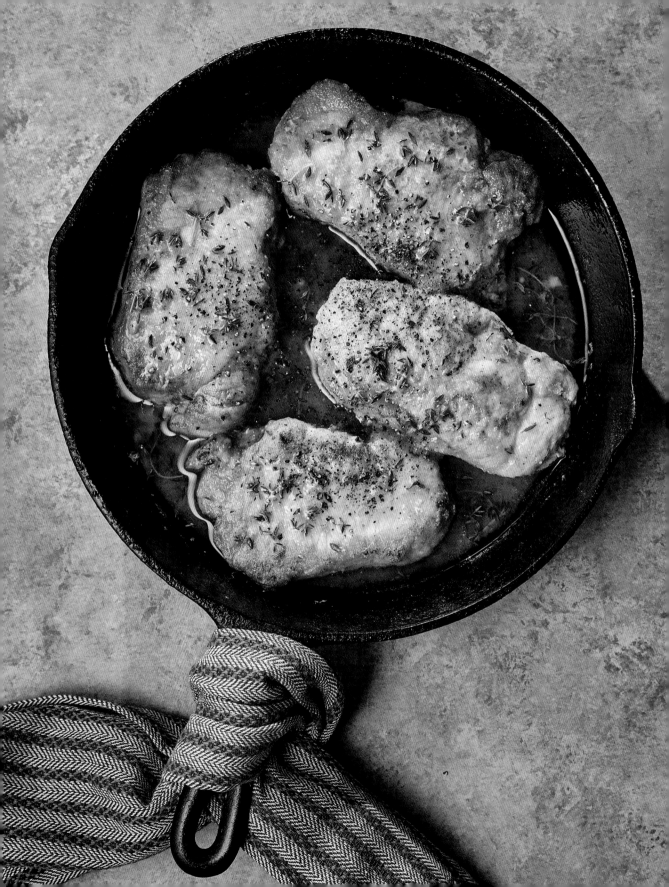

Creamy Lemon Thyme Pork Chops

YIELD: 4 SERVINGS

Pork chops can be dry and boring, but not these! They are juicy and have great fresh flavor from the thyme and lemon.

¼ cup (37 g) cassava flour

1 teaspoon salt

¼ teaspoon ground black pepper

4 pork chops, 1-inch (3 cm) thick (about 2 pounds [907 g])

2 tablespoons (30 ml) garlic-infused olive oil

Zest of 1 lemon

⅓ cup (80 ml) lemon juice

1 tablespoon (6 g) chopped fresh thyme

⅓ cup (80 g) ghee

Mix the cassava flour, salt, and pepper in a shallow bowl. Dredge the pork chops in the flour mixture, coating all sides. There may be some mixture left over.

Heat a large pan over medium heat and add the olive oil. Let it warm for 2 minutes. Add the pork chops and cook for 6 minutes without moving them. Flip and cook for 3 more minutes.

Transfer the pork chops to a plate. Add the lemon zest and juice, thyme, and ghee to the pan and cook for 2 minutes, or until a sauce is formed.

Add the pork chops back in and cook over low heat for 6–10 minutes, or until they reach 155°F (68°C) on a meat thermometer. Spoon the sauce over the pork chops as they cook.

Remove from the oven and serve immediately.

Store leftovers, covered, in the refrigerator for up to 6 days.

Apple Pork Chops

YIELD: 6 SERVINGS

Apple picking or just visiting the local farmers' market is one of my favorite fall activities. It usually results in lots of fresh apples and new ways to enjoy them. Pairing them with perfectly juicy pork chops is delicious. The apples are tender and sweet and add great autumn flavor to the dish. This is a light and flavorful meal that is sure to please.

PORK CHOPS

6 pork chops (2 pounds [907 g] total)

2 tablespoons (30 ml) melted ghee

2 teaspoons salt

1 teaspoon dried sage

APPLE TOPPING

2 medium apples, cored and sliced

1 tablespoon (15 g) ghee

⅛ teaspoon salt

½ teaspoon ground cinnamon

2 tablespoons (30 ml) water (optional)

Preheat the oven to 400°F (200°C or gas mark 6). Line a baking sheet with parchment paper.

Make the pork chops: Place the pork chops on the prepared baking sheet, brush with the ghee on both sides, and sprinkle with the salt and sage.

Bake for 20–25 minutes, or until the pork reaches 145°F (63°C) on a meat thermometer.

While the pork chops cook, make the apple topping: Place the apples, ghee, salt, and cinnamon in a large skillet over medium heat and cook for 8–10 minutes. Add the water if needed to prevent sticking during cooking.

Transfer the pork chops to a platter and ladle the apples over them to serve.

Store leftovers, covered, in the refrigerator for up to 6 days.

Pork Rind–Crusted Pork Chops

YIELD: 2 SERVINGS

If you are looking for a crunchy coated pork chop, this is it! The pork rinds crisp up so nicely and make the most amazing crust.

2 tablespoons (30 ml) melted ghee

2 ounces (57 g) plain pork rinds, blended or crushed until fine (look for humanely raised pork rinds, such as Epic or 4505)

½ teaspoon salt

¼ teaspoon ground black pepper

2 pork chops, 1-inch (3 cm) thick (1 pound [454 g] total)

Preheat the oven to 400°F (200°C or gas mark 6). Line a rimmed baking sheet with parchment paper. Put a wire rack on top of the baking sheet. This will help keep the pork chops crispy as they cook.

Place the melted ghee in a shallow dish and the pork rinds in a separate shallow dish along with the salt and pepper. Dip the pork chops in the ghee, coating fully, then in the pork rinds. Press the pork rinds into the chops to help them stick.

Place the pork chops on the wire rack and bake for 23–27 minutes, or until they reach 145°F (63°C) on a meat thermometer.

Remove from the oven and serve immediately.

Pecan–Crusted Chicken Tenders

YIELD: 4 SERVINGS

This tender chicken is coated in crunchy pecans that are baked to perfection. These will be loved by the whole family!

1¼ cups (140 g) finely chopped raw pecans

1 teaspoon salt

¼ teaspoon ground black pepper

1 teaspoon dried chives

1 tablespoon (15 ml) melted ghee

1 tablespoon (15 ml) garlic-infused olive oil

1–1¼ pounds (454–567 kg) chicken tenders or breasts cut into strips

Preheat the oven to 400°F (200°C or gas mark 6). Line a baking sheet with parchment paper and then place a wire rack on top. This will help the chicken stay crispy.

Place the pecans in a shallow dish and add the salt, pepper, and chives. Mix well.

In a separate shallow dish, combine the melted ghee and olive oil.

Dip the chicken pieces into the ghee mixture and then into the pecan mixture. Press the pecans onto the chicken so they adhere. Place on the wire rack on the prepared baking sheet.

Repeat with the remaining chicken.

Bake for 14–17 minutes, or until the coating is crisp and golden.

Remove from the oven and serve immediately. They are great by themselves but you can also use paleo ranch dressing as a dip.

Store leftovers, covered, in the refrigerator for up to 6 days.

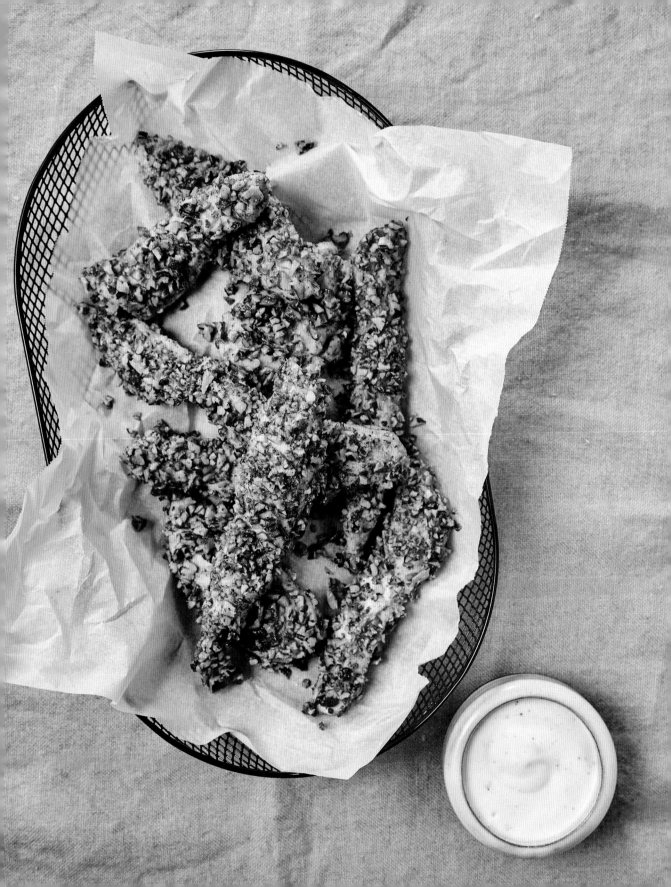

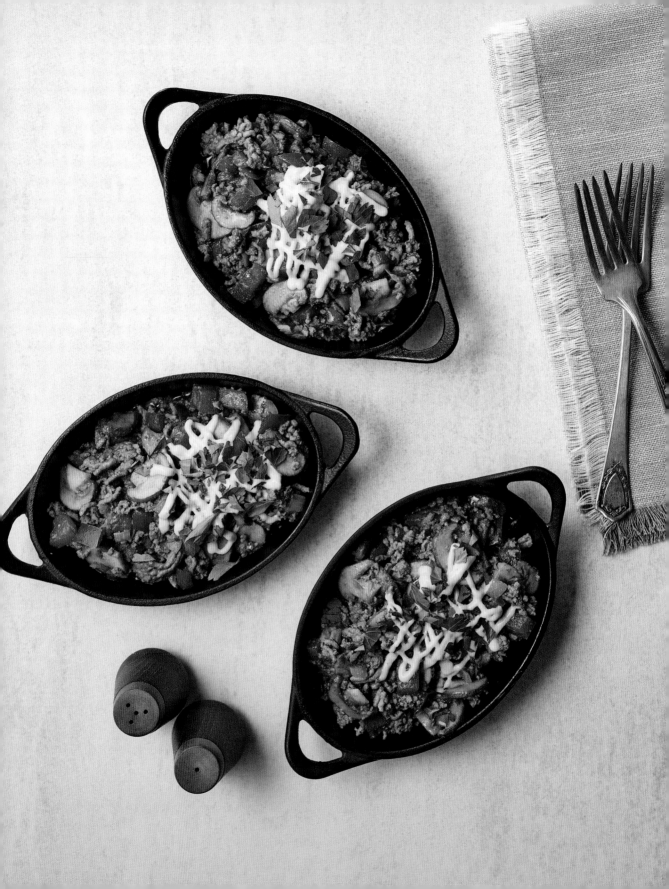

Philly Cheesesteak Skillet

YIELD: 6 TO 8 SERVINGS

Using ground beef is a shortcut that makes this dish come together quickly. The mayo topping is in place of the traditional cheese and adds great creaminess.

SKILLET

2 tablespoons (30 ml) avocado oil

1 large onion, chopped

1½ pounds (680 g) mushrooms, sliced

3 green peppers, cored and chopped

2 teaspoons (12 g) salt, divided

2 pounds (907 g) ground beef

2 tablespoons (30 ml) coconut aminos

1 teaspoon garlic powder

2 tablespoons (20 g) arrowroot powder/starch

TOPPING

1 cup (240 ml) paleo mayonnaise

2 tablespoons (30 ml) coconut aminos

¼ teaspoon garlic powder

¼ teaspoon onion powder

Make the skillet: Heat the avocado oil in a large skillet over medium heat. Add the onion, mushrooms, peppers, and 1 teaspoon of the salt and cook, stirring regularly, for 10 minutes.

Add the ground beef, remaining 1 teaspoon salt, coconut aminos, and garlic powder. Cook for 10–15 minutes, or until the meat is fully cooked and the vegetables are tender. Sprinkle in the arrowroot powder and stir well for 3–5 minutes, or until thick.

Make the topping: Combine the mayonnaise, coconut aminos, garlic powder, and onion powder in a small bowl. Drizzle over the skillet when serving.

Cabbage Sausage Skillet

YIELD: 6 SERVINGS

This simple meal comes together quickly. It is flavorful and filling, and the sauce pairs perfectly with the cabbage and sausage.

PALEO SIMPLE

CABBAGE AND SAUSAGE

1 tablespoon (15 ml) avocado oil

12 ounces (340 g) sugar-free kielbasa (such as Pederson's Farms), sliced into ½-inch (1 cm) slices

1 onion, diced

3 cloves garlic, minced

½ teaspoon salt

1 large head cabbage (about 3 pounds [1.4 kg]), chopped

SAUCE

2 tablespoons (30 g) spicy brown mustard

1 tablespoon (15 ml) apple cider vinegar

¼ cup (60 ml) olive oil

¼ teaspoon ground black pepper

½ teaspoon garlic powder

Heat the avocado oil in a large skillet over medium heat. Add the sausage and cook, stirring regularly, for 5 minutes. Add the onion, garlic, and salt and cook, stirring regularly, for 5 more minutes.

Add the cabbage, in portions if the pan isn't big enough, and cook, stirring regularly, for 15–20 minutes, or until the cabbage is tender.

While the cabbage is cooking, make the sauce: Combine the mustard, vinegar, olive oil, pepper, and garlic powder in a small bowl. Mix well.

Turn off the heat and stir the sauce into the cabbage mixture. Serve immediately.

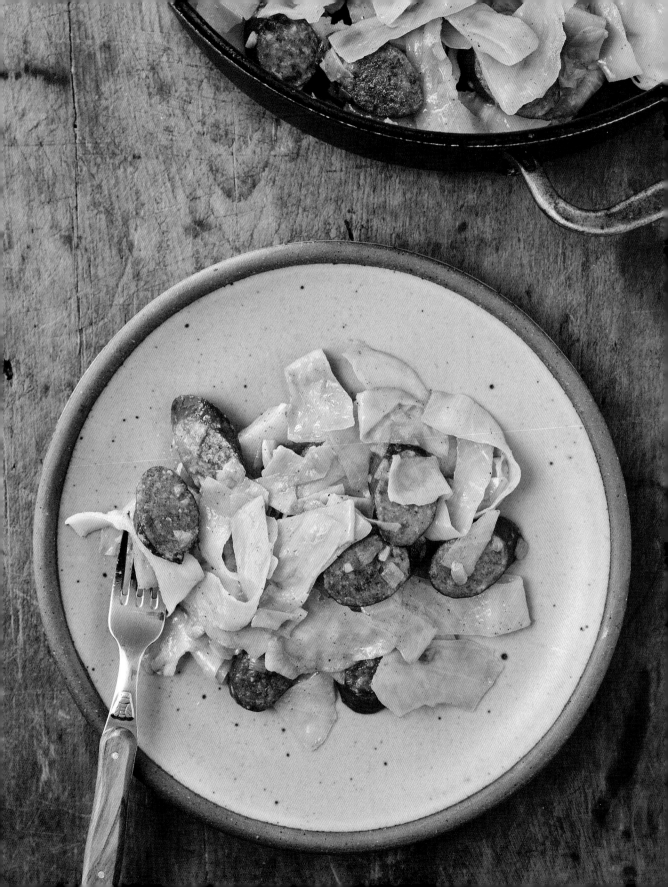

Creamy Cajun Chicken over Zucchini Noodles

YIELD: 6 TO 8 SERVINGS

Chicken thighs and sausage combine with a zesty sauce for one incredible meal. It's a little smoky and has just a little spice.

2 tablespoons (30 ml) avocado oil

2 bell peppers, cored and diced

1 large onion, diced

6 boneless skinless chicken thighs, cut into ½-inch (1 cm) pieces

12 ounces (340 g) andouille sausage (I use Pederson's), sliced into ½-inch (1 cm) pieces

One 13.5-ounce (378 ml) can full-fat coconut milk

3 or 4 medium zucchini, spiralized

Heat the avocado oil in a large skillet over medium heat. Add the bell peppers and onion and cook for 5-7 minutes, or until the veggies start to get tender.

Add the chicken thighs and cook for 5 minutes. Add the sausage and cook for 3 minutes.

Add the coconut milk and cook for 5 minutes, or until warmed. Serve over the zucchini noodles or stir the zucchini noodles into the sauce.

Store leftovers, covered, in the refrigerator for up to 6 days.

Egg Roll Meatballs

YIELD: 4 SERVINGS

All the flavors of an egg roll, packed into bite-size meatballs! Adding veggies to the meat helps bulk up the mixture and gives them great texture. The ginger, sesame oil, and coconut aminos give them an Asian-inspired taste that will satisfy any take-out craving.

One 14-ounce (392 g) bag coleslaw mix, divided

½ cup (64 g) shredded carrot

1-inch (3 cm) piece fresh ginger, peeled and grated

½ cup (64 g) diced onion

1 teaspoon salt

3 tablespoons (45 ml) coconut aminos

1 tablespoon (15 ml) toasted sesame oil

1 teaspoon garlic powder

1 pound (454 g) ground turkey or pork

Preheat the oven to 400°F (200°C or gas mark 6). Line a baking sheet with parchment paper.

Place 3 cups (180 g) of the coleslaw mix, carrot, ginger, and onion in a food processor and blend for less than 1 minute, or until the vegetables are very small and equal in size.

Transfer the veggie mixture to a large skillet over medium heat. Add the salt, coconut aminos, sesame oil, and garlic powder. Cook for 5 minutes, or until the vegetables are tender.

Transfer the veggie mixture to a large bowl. Add the ground turkey and mix well.

Roll into twenty-four 1-inch (3 cm) balls, arrange on the prepared baking sheet, and bake for 20 minutes.

Serve with the remaining coleslaw mix, if desired.

Store leftovers, covered, in the refrigerator for up to a week.

Chicken Alfredo–Stuffed Potatoes

YIELD: 6 TO 8 SERVINGS

This creamy chicken Alfredo and perfectly cooked broccoli are served on a baked sweet potato. The potatoes can be made ahead, making it a great weeknight meal. You could also serve chicken Alfredo over baked white potatoes instead of sweet potatoes if you prefer.

6 medium sweet potatoes

ALFREDO SAUCE

2 tablespoons (30 ml) garlic-infused olive oil

2 tablespoons (30 g) ghee

1 heaping tablespoon (10 g) arrowroot powder

2½ cups (600 ml) almond milk

½ teaspoon salt

¼ teaspoon ground black pepper

2 tablespoons (6 g) chopped fresh chives

CHICKEN

1 tablespoon (15 ml) garlic-infused olive oil

1½–2 pounds (680–907 g) boneless skinless chicken, cut into 1-inch (3 cm) pieces

1 teaspoon salt

BROCCOLI

2 tablespoons (30 g) ghee

One 10-ounce (283 g) bag frozen broccoli

¼ teaspoon salt

Preheat the oven to 400°F (200°C or gas mark 6). Line a baking sheet with parchment paper.

Wash and dry the sweet potatoes and place them on the prepared baking sheet. Bake for 40–50 minutes, or until fork tender.

While the potatoes cook, make the sauce: Heat the olive oil and ghee in a large saucepan over medium heat. Whisk in the arrowroot powder until fully combined. Add the almond milk and whisk for about 4 minutes, or until the mixture is smooth and thick. Add the salt, pepper, and chives. Leave in the pan until needed or pour into a bowl if you need the pan for the chicken.

Make the chicken: Heat the olive oil in a large skillet over medium heat. Add the chicken and salt and cook for 5–7 minutes, or until the chicken is cooked through. Add the chicken to the sauce.

Make the broccoli: Heat the ghee in a large skillet over medium heat, add the broccoli and salt, and cook, breaking the big pieces up with a spatula, for 5–7 minutes. Add to the chicken mixture and stir.

Remove the potatoes from the oven and cut them in half. Spoon the chicken Alfredo over the potatoes. Serve warm.

Asian Chicken Thighs

YIELD: 6 TO 8 SERVINGS

These tender, juicy chicken thighs are coated in a savory sauce. They come together quickly and make a great weeknight meal. It's simple, but so satisfying.

6–8 bone-in skin-on chicken thighs (about 3½ pounds [1.6 kg])

¼ cup (60 ml) coconut aminos

1 tablespoon (15 ml) toasted sesame oil

1 tablespoon (15 ml) garlic-infused olive oil

1 tablespoon (15 g) peeled and grated fresh ginger

½ teaspoon red pepper flakes

1¼ teaspoons (7.5 g) salt

Preheat the oven to 400°F (200°C or gas mark 6). Place the chicken thighs in a 13 by 9-inch (33 by 23 cm) pan.

Combine the coconut aminos, sesame oil, olive oil, ginger, and red pepper flakes in a small bowl. Stir and pour over the chicken. Sprinkle the salt evenly on top of the chicken thighs.

Bake for 45 minutes, or until the chicken reaches 165°F (74°C) on a meat thermometer.

Serve with the sauce scooped over the chicken.

Store leftovers, covered, in the refrigerator for up to 6 days.

Hamburger Stroganoff

YIELD: 6 TO 8 SERVINGS

This stroganoff features a rich, silky sauce filled with mushrooms and ground beef. This is a no-fuss meal that is sure to be loved. It's great served over zucchini noodles or mashed potatoes!

2 tablespoons (30 ml) avocado oil

½ large onion, diced (1½ cups [192 g])

4 cloves garlic, minced

2 pounds (907 g) ground beef

2 teaspoons (12 g) salt

1 pound (454 g) mushrooms, sliced

¼ cup (60 ml) coconut aminos

1 cup (240 ml) full-fat coconut milk

2 tablespoons (20 g) arrowroot powder/starch

1 teaspoon dried thyme

1 teaspoon mild paprika

½ teaspoon ground black pepper

Heat the avocado oil in a large skillet over medium heat. Add the onion and garlic and cook for 5 minutes.

Add the beef and salt and cook, stirring regularly, for 5 minutes. Add the mushrooms and coconut aminos and cook for 5 minutes, or until the mushrooms start to soften.

Combine the coconut milk and arrowroot powder in a small bowl and add to the skillet. Cook for about 3 minutes, or until thick.

Add the thyme, paprika, and pepper and stir well. Serve immediately.

Store leftovers, covered, in the refrigerator for up to 6 days.

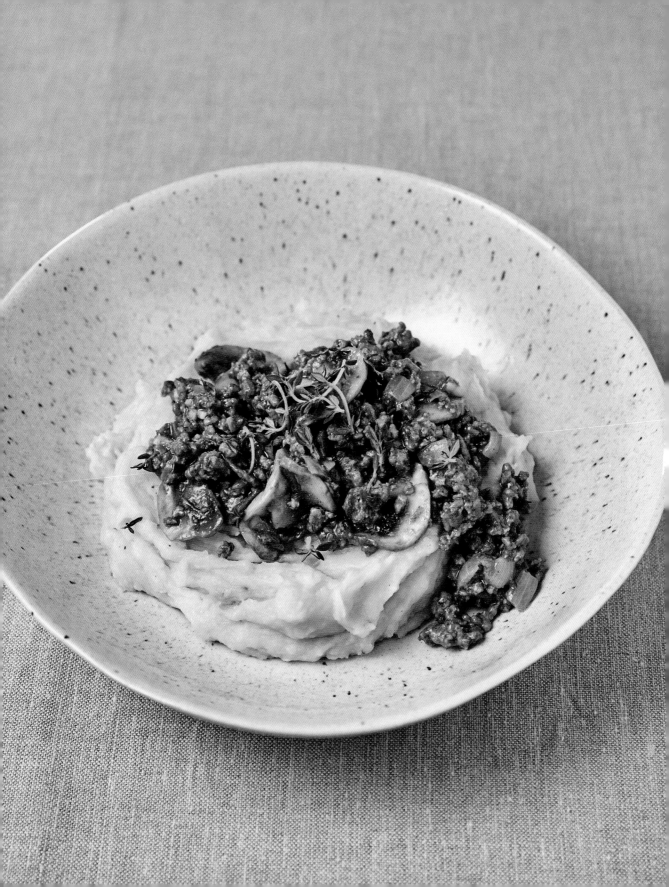

Mexican Skillet

YIELD: 4 SERVINGS

This is a hearty one-pan meal loaded with spice. The perfectly cooked sweet potatoes balance out the savory seasonings.

1 tablespoon (15 ml) avocado oil

½ large onion, diced

1 bell pepper, cored and chopped

1 pound (454 g) ground beef

½ teaspoon salt

½ teaspoon ground black pepper

1 tablespoon (6 g) chili powder

1 teaspoon ground cumin

1 teaspoon paprika

1 teaspoon dried oregano

One 4-ounce (113 g) can diced green chiles

One 14.5-ounce (411 g) can fire-roasted diced tomatoes

½ cup (120 ml) water

1 pound (454 g) sweet potatoes, chopped into ½-inch (1 cm) pieces

Heat the avocado oil in a large skillet over medium heat. Add the onion and bell pepper and cook for 5 minutes. Add the beef and salt and cook, breaking up the beef with a wooden spoon, for 3 minutes.

Add the black pepper, chili powder, cumin, paprika, oregano, green chiles, tomatoes, water, and sweet potatoes. Stir well, cover, and cook over medium heat for 15 minutes, or until the potatoes are tender.

Remove from the heat and serve immediately.

Store leftovers, covered, in the refrigerator for up to 6 days.

Chili Dog Casserole

YIELD: 8 TO 10 SERVINGS

This is a fun and pleasing meal the whole family will love. Chili and hot dogs make the first layer, topped with creamy mashed potatoes.

BEEF LAYER

1 pound (454 g) ground beef

1 teaspoon salt

1 large onion, diced

4 cloves garlic, minced

One 25-ounce (709 g) can crushed tomatoes

One 14.5-ounce (411 g) can diced tomatoes

¼ cup (24 g) chili powder

6 nitrate-free hot dogs (such as Teton Water Ranch or Applegate), cut into ½-inch (1 cm) slices

MASHED POTATO TOPPING

3 pounds (1.4 kg) Yukon gold potatoes

½ teaspoon salt

1 cup (240 ml) chicken broth

½ teaspoon garlic powder

¼ teaspoon ground black pepper

Make the beef mixture: Place the beef and salt in a large skillet and cook over medium heat, breaking it apart as it cooks, for 5 minutes.

Add the onion and garlic and cook for 5 minutes.

Add the tomatoes, chili powder, and hot dogs and cook over low heat for 20–30 minutes.

While the beef mixture cooks, make the mashed potatoes: Wash and cut the potatoes into fourths. Place the potatoes in a 2-quart (2 L) pot, cover with cold water, and add the salt. Turn the heat to medium-high and stir occasionally until the water boils. This should take 8–10 minutes.

Cover, turn the heat to low, and cook for 10–15 minutes, or until a fork can easily pierce a potato.

Turn off the heat, drain the potatoes, and return them to the hot pot. Add the chicken broth, garlic powder, and pepper and mash with a potato masher until smooth.

Preheat the oven to 375°F (190°C or gas mark 5). Line a 13 by 9-inch (33 by 23 cm) pan with parchment paper or grease well with coconut oil.

Place the chili dog mixture in the bottom of the prepared pan and top evenly with the mashed potatoes, spreading them to the edges. Bake for 30 minutes.

Remove from the oven and serve immediately.

Store leftovers, covered, in the refrigerator for up to 6 days.

Korean Shredded Beef

This beef has Asian flair from the ginger, sesame oil, and coconut aminos. It's bursting with flavor and so tender and delicious. Serve over a bowl of greens or in grain-free tortillas.

1-1¼ pounds (454-568 g) flank steak, cut against the grain into fourths

¼ cup (60 ml) coconut aminos

2 teaspoons (10 ml) toasted sesame oil

½ large onion, chopped

3 cloves garlic, minced

1 teaspoon ground ginger

½ teaspoon red pepper flakes

¼ teaspoon salt

Place the beef in the electric pressure cooker. Add the coconut aminos, sesame oil, onion, garlic, ginger, red pepper flakes, and salt. Stir to combine.

Place the lid on, close the valve, and cook on High for 40 minutes. Let naturally release for 15 minutes; this helps the meat stay juicy.

Press Cancel, release the valve, and open the lid. Press Sauté and cook, stirring to help shred the meat, for 8-10 minutes. The juices should reduce. Serve immediately.

Store leftovers, covered, in the refrigerator for up to a week.

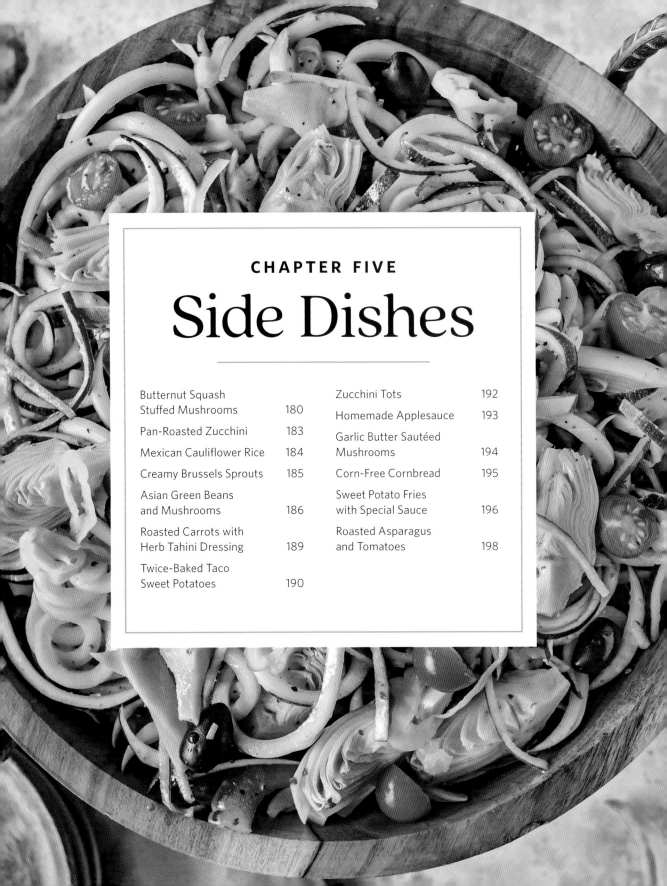

Butternut Squash Stuffed Mushrooms

YIELD: 4 SERVINGS

These stuffed portobello mushrooms make me think that I could try being a vegetarian again. Just kidding. Truly, though, these creamy and savory stuffed mushrooms are the perfect complement to your dinner. The slightly sweet squash has a hint of anise flavor, the mushrooms are spiked with garlic and thyme, and it's all topped off with some tangy sun-dried tomatoes and goat cheese. You might just want to have two and call it a meal!

SQUASH

2 cups (300 g) ½-inch (1.3 cm) diced butternut squash

1 tablespoon (15 ml) extra virgin olive oil

1 tablespoon (9 g) coconut sugar

1 heaping teaspoon (2 g) fennel seeds

Kosher salt, to taste

Black pepper, to taste

MUSHROOMS

4 cloves garlic, minced

2 tablespoons (30 ml) extra virgin olive oil

1 tablespoon (2.4 g) fresh thyme leaves, coarsely chopped

4 portobello mushroom caps, gills removed and wiped clean

FILLING

¼ cup (27.5 g) sun-dried tomatoes in oil, drained and finely chopped

¼ cup (40 g) gluten-free bread crumbs

¼ cup (37 g) crumbled goat cheese

Arugula, for serving

Fresh lemon juice, for serving

Extra virgin olive oil, for serving

Balsamic vinegar, for serving

Preheat the oven to 400°F (200°C or gas mark 6). Adjust the oven rack to the middle position and line a baking sheet with parchment paper.

To make the squash, in a large bowl, toss together the squash, olive oil, coconut sugar, fennel seeds, and a big pinch of salt and pepper. Use your hands to toss until everything is combined. Transfer the squash to the prepared baking sheet and roast until golden, 15 to 20 minutes.

When finished, remove from the oven and reduce the temperature to 375°F (190°C or gas mark 5). Line a new baking sheet with parchment paper.

Meanwhile, to make the mushrooms, combine the garlic, olive oil, and thyme in a small bowl. Brush the inside of each mushroom cap with this mixture.

To make the filling, in the same bowl, combine the sun-dried tomatoes and bread crumbs.

Divide the squash evenly among the mushroom caps. Top them with the tomato and bread crumb mixture. Dollop a few chunks of goat cheese on each and place on the new baking sheet.

Bake until the mushrooms become tender and the tops turn golden brown, 12 to 16 minutes.

To serve, lay each mushroom on a bed of baby arugula and drizzle with lemon juice, olive oil, and vinegar.

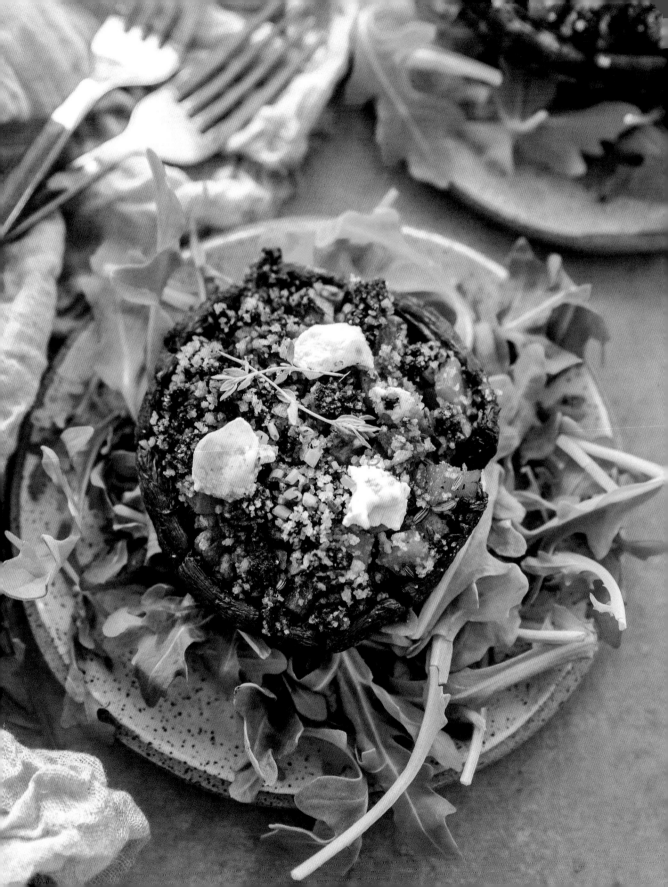

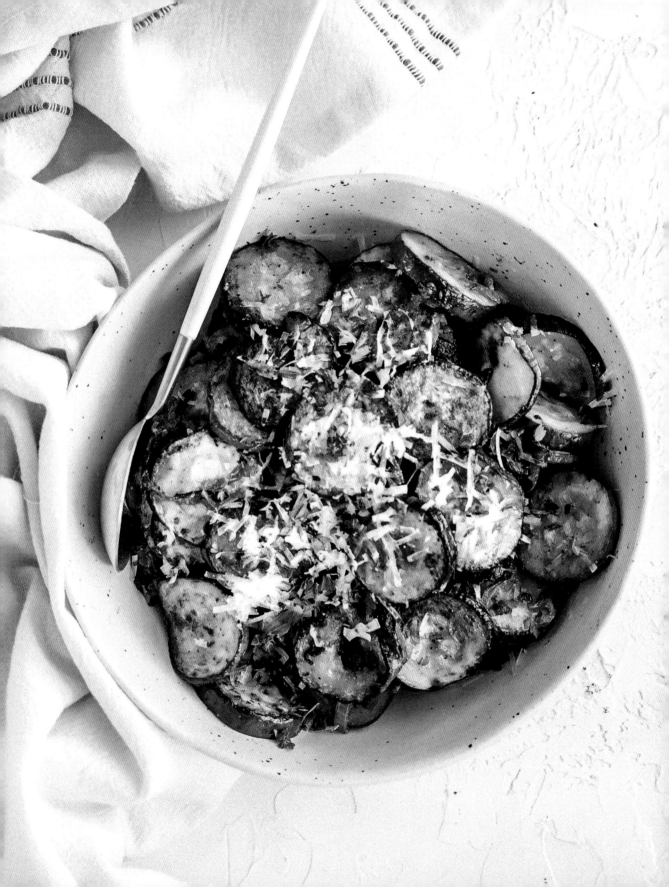

Pan-Roasted Zucchini

YIELD: 4 SERVINGS

There's nothing quite like a straightforward but flavorful side dish like this pan-roasted zucchini. It takes very little time to prepare and almost no time on the stove at all. You can have everything done in less than twenty minutes, and it tastes absolutely divine with the grated Parmesan on top.

3 tablespoons (45 ml) avocado oil, divided

½ yellow onion, sliced

4 medium zucchini (about 2 pounds [900 g]), cut into ½-inch (1.3 cm) rounds

1 teaspoon (6 g) kosher salt, plus more to taste

½ teaspoon garlic powder

¼ teaspoon black pepper, plus more to taste

3 tablespoons (45 ml) chicken bone broth

¼ cup (22 g) grated Parmesan cheese

In a large skillet, heat 1 ½ tablespoons (22 ml) of the oil for 2 minutes over medium heat. Add the onion and cook until soft, 4 to 5 minutes.

Add the zucchini, salt, garlic powder, and pepper. Cook, stirring frequently, until softened, about 7 minutes. Add the broth and cook until the broth has evaporated, 2 to 3 minutes more. Add the remaining 1½ tablespoons (22 ml) oil and cook for another few minutes, until the zucchini browns on the edges.

Remove from the heat and sprinkle with the Parmesan. Taste and add salt and pepper as needed.

SIDE DISHES

Mexican Cauliflower Rice

YIELD: 4 SERVINGS

This super-easy, Mexican-inspired cauliflower rice is a must for your next Taco Tuesday. It's infused with amazing Mexican flavors, such as paprika, cumin, jalapeño, and cilantro.

1 large head cauliflower, trimmed and cut into florets (see Note)

1 tablespoon (15 ml) olive oil

½ medium yellow onion, diced

1 jalapeño, seeded and sliced (optional)

2 cloves garlic, minced

⅓ cup (80 ml) compliant beef broth

3½ tablespoons (52 g) tomato paste

Juice of ½ lime

1 teaspoon ground cumin

½ teaspoon paprika

Sea salt and black pepper to taste

Chopped cilantro, for garnish

Add the cauliflower florets to a food processor. Pulse until the cauliflower resembles small rice-like bits. Make sure not to overpulse.

Heat the olive oil in a large skillet over medium heat, then add the onion, jalapeño (if using), and garlic.

Add the riced cauliflower and cook until tender, about 4 minutes.

In a separate bowl, whisk together the broth, tomato paste, and lime juice. Pour into the skillet and stir to combine.

Season with the cumin, paprika, and a pinch of salt and pepper. Taste and add more salt and pepper, if necessary.

Garnish with the cilantro before serving.

Note

You can buy cauliflower rice pretty much everywhere these days (though it's expensive!). If you go that route, use about 5 cups (700 g) for this recipe.

Creamy Brussels Sprouts

YIELD: 5 OR 6 SERVINGS

If you haven't been a fan of Brussels sprouts before, you're in for a surprise. And if you do like them, well, you're in for a real treat. Here, I add flavor to plain sprouts by cooking them in a cream sauce and topping with crumbled bacon. You'll want to keep this dish all to yourself.

3 slices compliant bacon

1½ tablespoons (23 ml) olive oil

2 small shallots, diced

2 cloves garlic, minced

2 pounds (910 g) Brussels sprouts, trimmed and halved

1 cup (240 ml) canned unsweetened coconut milk

¼ cup (60 ml) no sugar added beef broth

1 tablespoon (4 g) nutritional yeast

1 teaspoon crushed red pepper flakes

Sea salt and black pepper, to taste

1½ teaspoons tapioca flour or arrowroot powder, dissolved in 2 teaspoons water

Preheat the oven to 400°F (200°C or gas mark 6).

Place the bacon on a baking sheet. Bake until the desired doneness, 15 to 20 minutes.

Transfer the cooked bacon to a paper towel to drain the excess oil. Chop when cool.

Meanwhile, heat the olive oil in a large skillet over medium-high heat. Add the shallots and garlic and cook, stirring frequently, until fragrant and tender, 1 to 2 minutes.

Add the Brussels sprouts. Cook, stirring occasionally, until tender, 8 to 10 minutes.

Add the coconut milk, broth, nutritional yeast, red pepper flakes, and a generous pinch of salt and pepper. Stir together with a spoon until all the ingredients are combined.

Add the tapioca mixture. Turn the heat to low and cook until the sauce thickens, 4 to 5 minutes more.

Crumble the bacon over the top of the Brussels sprouts before serving.

Asian Green Beans and Mushrooms

YIELD: 4 SERVINGS

Green beans and mushrooms are the new peas and carrots. When cooked in coconut aminos, rice vinegar, sesame oil, ginger, and garlic, they're perfect to serve with chicken or a paleo-inspired main dish.

1 pound (454 g) fresh green beans, trimmed

1 tablespoon (14 g) ghee

2 cloves garlic, minced

1½ cups (105 g) button mushrooms

¼ cup (60 ml) coconut aminos

1 tablespoon (15 ml) sesame oil

1 tablespoon (15 ml) rice vinegar

¼ teaspoon ground ginger

Sesame seeds, for garnish

Prepare a large bowl of ice and water.

Bring a pot of water to a boil and blanch the green beans until they are bright green, about 2 minutes. Immediately transfer the green beans to the ice water.

Once the green beans are cool, drain and pat dry using a dish towel.

Heat the ghee in a large skillet over medium heat until the ghee sizzles. Add the garlic and stir for about 30 seconds.

Add the mushrooms and cook until tender, 2 to 3 minutes.

Transfer the green beans to the skillet and toss together. Cook for 5 minutes.

In a small bowl, whisk together the coconut aminos, sesame oil, vinegar, and ginger.

Reduce the heat to low and add the liquid mixture to the skillet. Stir well and simmer for 1 to 2 minutes more.

Sprinkle with the sesame seeds and serve immediately.

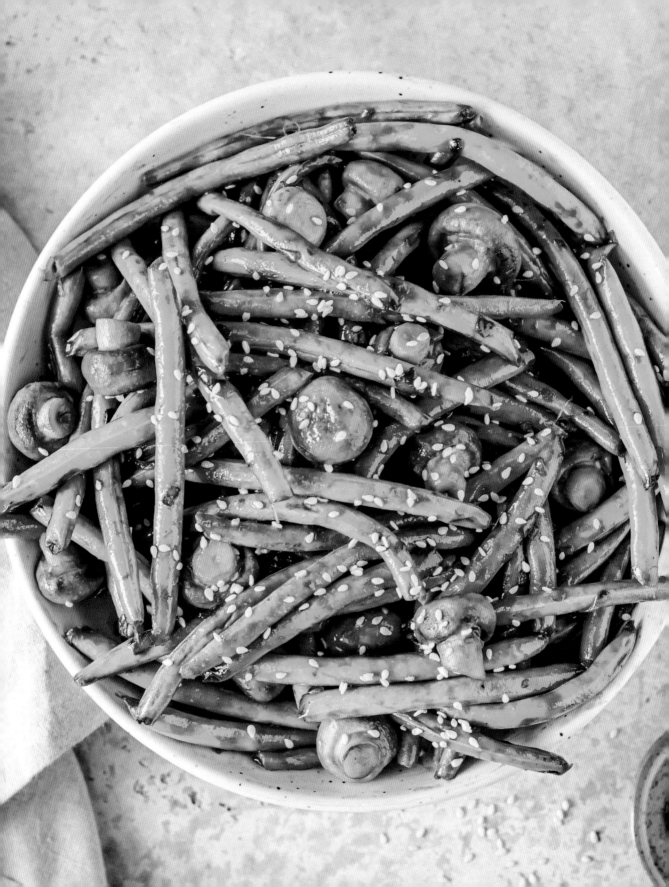

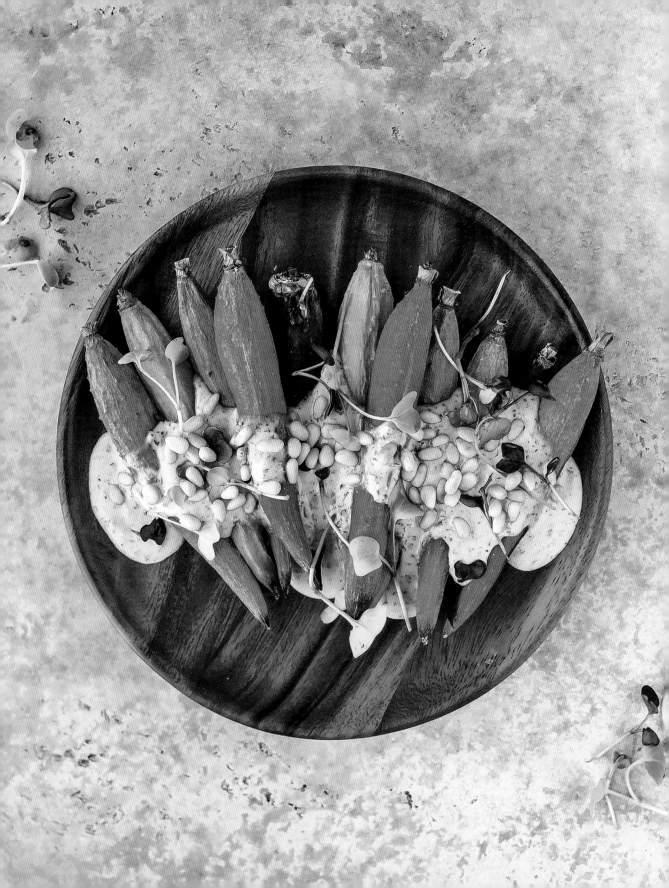

Roasted Carrots
with Herb Tahini Dressing

YIELD: 4 SERVINGS

These pretty roasted carrots, drizzled with an herbed tahini sauce, are the perfect side to chicken, pork, or steak.

ROASTED CARROTS

1 large bunch rainbow carrots, scrubbed

1 tablespoon (15 ml) olive oil

½ teaspoon sea salt

2 tablespoons (16 g) pine nuts

Microgreens, for garnish (optional)

HERB TAHINI DRESSING

¼ cup (60 g) tahini

¼ cup (60 ml) water

Juice of 1 lemon

¼ cup (16 g) chopped fresh parsley

¼ cup (10 g) chopped fresh basil

2 tablespoons (6 g) chopped chives

1 clove garlic

Sea salt and black pepper, to taste

Roasted carrots

Preheat the oven to 425°F (220°C or gas mark 7). Oil a baking sheet.

Place the carrots on the baking sheet. Drizzle with the olive oil and sprinkle with the salt. Toss to coat the carrots.

Roast until the carrots are tender and golden, about 20 minutes.

Remove the carrots from the oven and transfer to a plate.

Drizzle with 2 to 3 tablespoons (30 to 45 ml) of the Herb Tahini Dressing and sprinkle with the pine nuts. Garnish with microgreens, if desired.

Herb tahini dressing

Add the olive oil, tahini, water, lemon juice, parsley, basil, chives, garlic, and a pinch of salt and pepper to a high-speed blender or food processor. Blend until smooth, about 1 minute.

If the mixture is too thick, add a little more water. Taste and add more salt and pepper, if necessary.

Add any extra dressing to a mason jar and cap it with a lid. Will keep for up to 1 week in the fridge.

Twice-Baked Taco Sweet Potatoes

YIELD: 8 SERVINGS

These twice-baked sweet potatoes are filled with all the flavors of Taco Tuesday. They can be served not only as an appetizer but also as a main dish.

4 large sweet potatoes, scrubbed

1 tablespoon (15 ml) olive oil

¼ cup (40 g) chopped onion

1 pound (454 g) 90/10 ground beef

2 tablespoons (30 ml) canned unsweetened coconut milk

2 tablespoons (8 g) nutritional yeast

1¼ teaspoons chili powder

1 teaspoon ground cumin

½ teaspoon onion powder

½ teaspoon garlic powder

¼ teaspoon dried oregano

¼ teaspoon sea salt

1 avocado, peeled, pitted, and diced, for garnish

Compliant salsa, for garnish

Preheat the oven to 375°F (190°C or gas mark 5). Pierce the potatoes several times with a fork. Set on a baking sheet and bake until tender, about 60 minutes.

Meanwhile, heat the olive oil in a large skillet over medium-high heat. Add the onion and cook until translucent, 4 to 5 minutes. Add the ground beef and cook until browned, 5 to 7 minutes.

Split the potatoes lengthwise and remove the insides of the sweet potatoes, transferring to a medium bowl. Reserve the skins for later.

To the flesh of the sweet potatoes, add the cooked ground beef and onions, along with the coconut milk, nutritional yeast, chili powder, cumin, onion powder, garlic powder, oregano, and salt. Mix together until completely combined.

Spoon the filling back into the potato skins and place on the baking sheet.

Return the potatoes to the oven and bake until golden brown, about 15 minutes.

Top each potato skin with avocado and salsa.

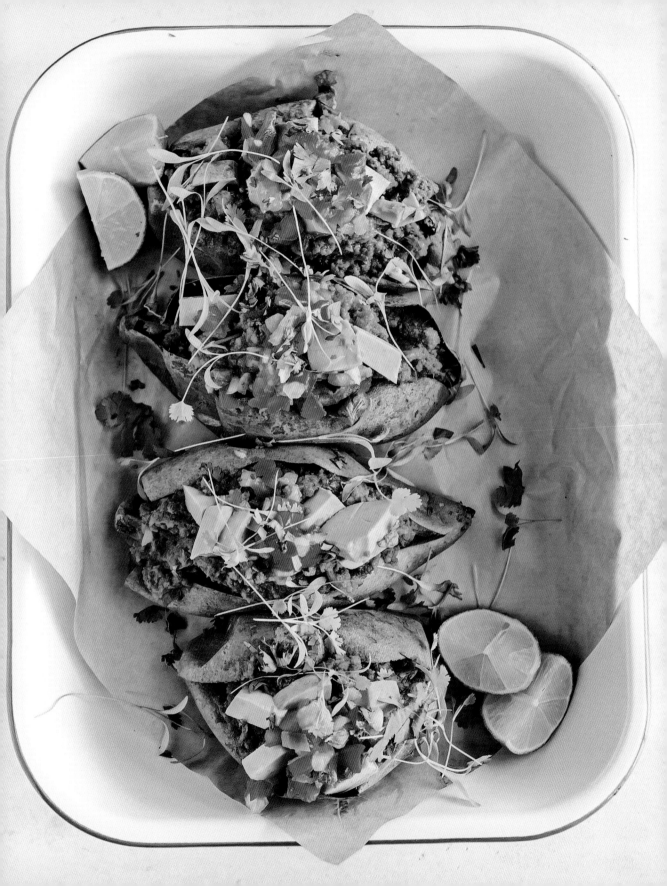

Zucchini Tots

Here's a fun way to eat zucchini. These are handheld and lightly seasoned, and make a great snack or side dish.

2 cups (248 g) packed shredded zucchini (about 2 medium zucchini)

1 large egg

3 tablespoons (23 g) coconut flour

½ teaspoon salt

¼ teaspoon ground black pepper

1 teaspoon Italian seasoning

1 tablespoon (15 ml) garlic-infused olive oil

Preheat the oven to 400°F (200°C or gas mark 6). Line a baking sheet with parchment paper.

Combine the zucchini, egg, coconut flour, salt, pepper, Italian seasoning, and oil in a large bowl. Mix with a wooden spoon until well combined.

Scoop into 1-tablespoon (15 g) balls and with your hands shape each into a tot shape, about 1½ inches (4 cm) long by 1 inch (3 cm) wide.

Bake for 12 minutes. Flip and bake for 12 more minutes. Bake for another 5 minutes if needed for tots to finish browning. Serve immediately. These are great dipped in paleo ranch dressing or marinara sauce.

Homemade Applesauce

YIELD: 8 TO 10 SERVINGS

This recipe is simple, but special. My family made this applesauce a lot while I was growing up, and it always tastes better than store-bought. No added sugar is needed, and I encourage you to try a bowl warm—it's delightful. Add a little cinnamon if you like, and use whatever apples you love. The pressure cooker version creates a thinner applesauce, whereas the stovetop version is thick and chunky.

3 pounds (1.4 kg) apples

½ cup (120 ml) water

Pressure cooker

Peel and core the apples and cut them into eighths. Place the apples pieces in the pressure cooker and add the water. Place the lid on and close the valve.

Cook on high for 8 minutes. Press Cancel and release the pressure. Press Sauté and cook for 3–5 minutes to thicken.

Stove

Peel and core the apples and cut them into eighths. Place the cut apples in a large saucepan. Add the water, cover, and cook, stirring every 10 minutes, for 30 minutes. Mash with a spoon or a potato masher.

Cook for another 10 minutes if you prefer a thicker sauce. Turn off the heat. Let cool for chunky applesauce; blend for smooth applesauce. You can do this with an immersion blender right in the pan or pour the mixture into a blender and blend until smooth.

Serve warm or store leftovers, covered, in the refrigerator for up to a week.

Garlic Butter Sautéed Mushrooms

YIELD: 4 SERVINGS

These mushrooms are quick to make and the perfect side to steak, chicken, or eggs. They are tender, flavorful, and the butter flavor comes from the ghee in this dish. The mushrooms can be prepped ahead and stored in the fridge if needed.

2 pounds (910 g) mushrooms, white or baby bellas

4 tablespoons (60 ml) ghee, divided

½ teaspoon salt

3 cloves minced garlic

1 tablespoon (2.4 g) fresh thyme

Wipe down the mushrooms with a damp cloth and cut into fourths.

Add 3 tablespoons (45 ml) of the ghee to a large skillet and turn heat to medium. Add in the mushrooms and cook for about 3 minutes, stirring to coat mushrooms in ghee. Let sit without stirring 7 minutes. During this time, the mushrooms will release a lot of moisture. Let that moisture cook off, stirring occasionally, which will take about 8 minutes.

Once the moisture has cooked off add the last tablespoon of ghee, garlic and thyme. Cook 2–3 minutes, until garlic is cooked and mushrooms are coated in the ghee.

PALEO SIMPLE

Corn-Free Cornbread

YIELD: 9 SERVINGS

It's amazing how much this cornbread tastes like the traditional version even though it doesn't use cornmeal. The almond flour and coconut flour mixture gives it that classic texture, and the honey gives it just the right amount of sweetness.

¾ cup (84 g) almond flour

¼ cup (30 g) coconut flour

¼ teaspoon salt

½ teaspoon baking soda

3 large eggs, at room temperature

¼ cup (60 ml) melted ghee

3 tablespoons (44 ml) honey

¼ cup (60 ml) almond milk

Preheat the oven to 350°F (180°C or gas mark 4). Line a 9 by 9-inch (23 by 23 cm) pan with parchment paper or grease well with coconut oil.

Combine the almond flour, coconut flour, salt, and baking soda in a large bowl. Mix well.

Add the eggs, ghee, honey, and almond milk and stir to combine.

Pour the mixture into the prepared pan and spread evenly. Bake for 25–28 minutes, or until the edges are golden brown. Serve warm. This is great with chili or soup.

Store leftovers, covered, at room temperature for up to 2 days or longer in the refrigerator.

Sweet Potato Fries with Special Sauce

YIELD: 3 TO 4 SERVINGS

These sweet potato fries are crispy thanks to the arrowroot powder and salting after baking. The sauce has a little spice that tastes amazing with the potatoes' sweetness.

1 large sweet potato

2 teaspoons (7 g) arrowroot powder/starch

1 tablespoon (15 ml) avocado oil

¼ teaspoon salt

SAUCE

⅓ cup (80 ml) paleo mayonnaise

¼ teaspoon chipotle powder

1 teaspoon garlic-infused olive oil

Preheat the oven to 425°F (220°C or gas mark 7). Line a baking sheet with parchment paper.

Cut the sweet potato into ¼-inch (6 mm) slices. (Note that I often like to cut the slices into ¼-inch [6 m] sticks.) Place them in a large bowl and toss with the arrowroot powder, trying to coat all the fries evenly. Leave any excess in the bowl. Arrange the fries in a single layer on the baking sheet. Drizzle with the avocado oil and toss to coat evenly. Do not salt at this point!

Bake for 15 minutes, remove from the oven and flip them, and then bake for another 15 minutes.

Remove from the oven and season with the salt.

Meanwhile, make the sauce: Place the mayo in a small bowl. Add the chipotle powder and olive oil. Stir well. Serve with the fries.

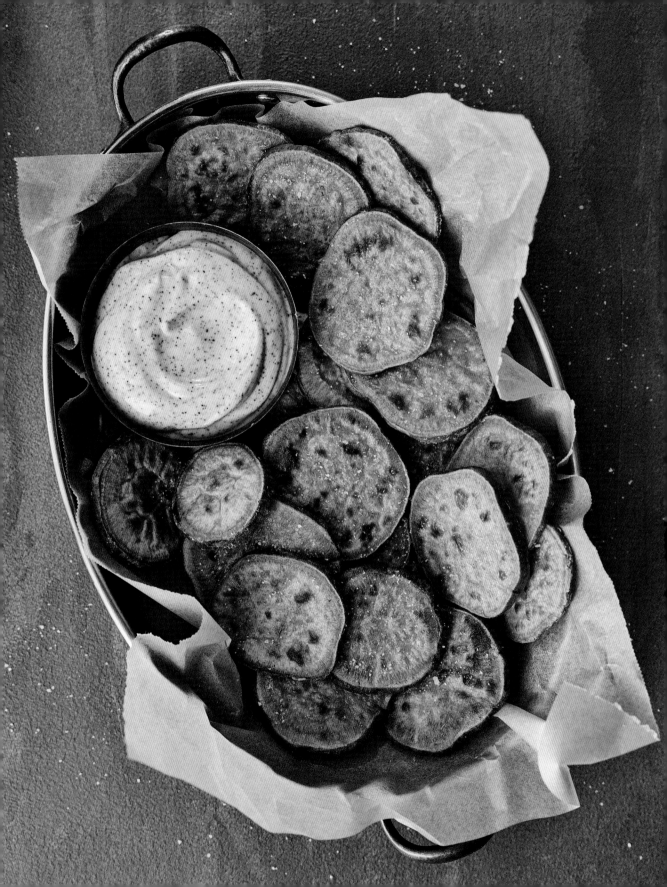

Roasted Asparagus and Tomatoes

YIELD: 4 SERVINGS

Plain roasted asparagus isn't that appetizing. However, this roasted asparagus with tomatoes, drizzled with a creamy lemon vinaigrette and topped with crunchy macadamia nuts, is both appetizing and delicious. This is a great side to serve with any protein, especially steak.

ASPARAGUS AND TOMATOES

1 bunch asparagus, ends trimmed

1½ cups (225 g) cherry tomatoes, halved

1½ tablespoons (23 ml) olive oil

¼ teaspoon sea salt

2 to 3 tablespoons (16 to 24 g) chopped macadamia nuts

LEMON VINAIGRETTE

3 tablespoons (45 ml) light olive oil

Juice of ½ lemon

½ teaspoon Dijon mustard

¼ teaspoon onion powder

⅛ teaspoon sea salt

Pinch of black pepper

Asparagus and tomatoes

Preheat the oven to 400°F (200°C or gas mark 6) and coat a baking sheet with olive oil cooking spray.

Arrange the asparagus on one end of the baking sheet and the tomatoes on the other. Drizzle with the olive oil and sprinkle with the salt.

Bake until the veggies soften and start to brown, 15 to 20 minutes.

Remove the sheet pan from the oven and place the asparagus and tomatoes on a large plate. Top with the lemon vinaigrette and macadamia nuts.

Lemon vinaigrette

In a small bowl, whisk together the olive oil, lemon juice, mustard, onion powder, salt, and pepper.

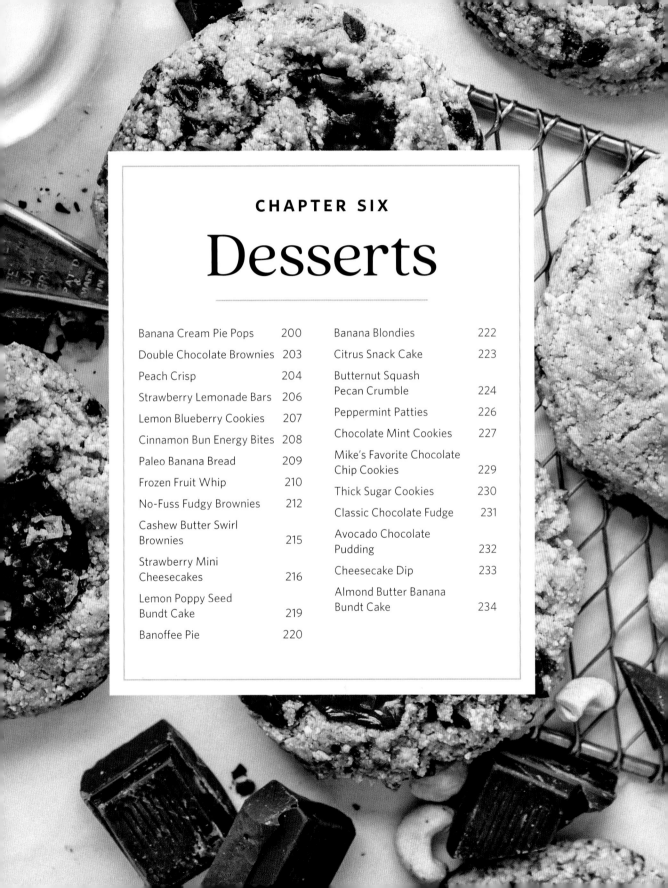

CHAPTER SIX

Desserts

Banana Cream Pie Pops

YIELD: 6 POPS

Growing up, banana cream pie was my favorite dessert. This ice-pop recipe plays on that, and it's perfect for all you banana lovers out there. Ice pops are a great way to tame a sweet tooth in a healthy and cool way.

1 whole banana

1 can (13.5 ounces [378 g]) unsweetened coconut milk

5 tablespoons (75 ml) sweetener of choice (I use maple syrup)

1 teaspoon pure vanilla extract

Pinch of sea salt

½ banana, sliced

6 ice-pop molds

⅓ cup (45 g) almonds

¼ cup (60 ml) pure maple syrup

Add the whole banana, coconut milk, sweetener, vanilla, and salt to a blender and blend until combined and smooth.

Place a couple of banana slices into each ice-pop mold.

Pour the creamy mixture into each ice-pop mold. Do not overfill it or the mixture will spill out the sides when putting on the lid.

Freeze until completely frozen, 2 to 3 hours.

Add the almonds to a food processor and pulse until ground.

Pour the maple syrup into a small bowl.

Remove the pops from the freezer and unmold. (You might have to quickly run them under warm water to loosen.)

Dip the tips of each pop into the maple syrup and then into the crushed almonds.

Serve immediately or return the ice pops to the freezer.

Note

Ice pops will keep for 3 or 4 weeks (without the syrup and almonds) if stored in an airtight container.

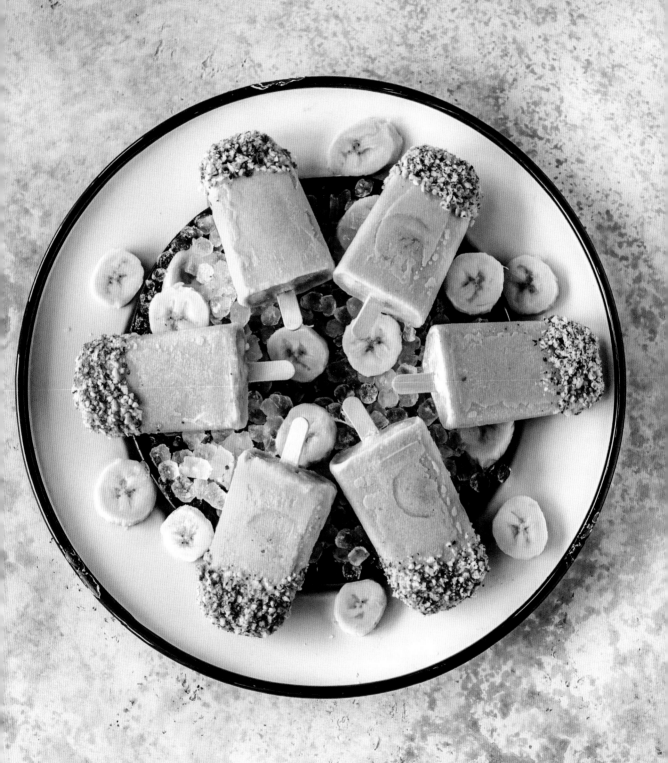

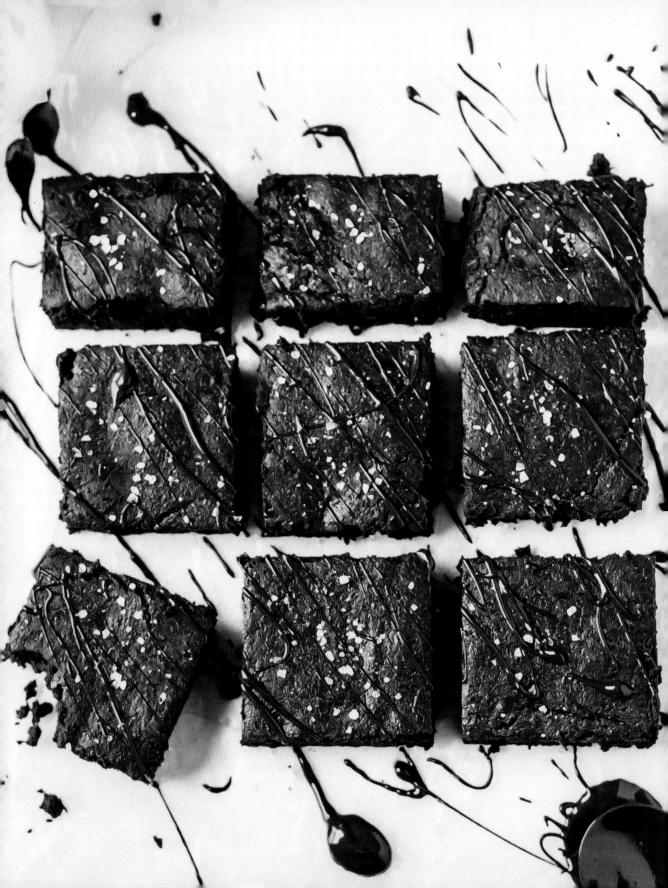

Double Chocolate Brownies

YIELD: 12 BROWNIES

Brownies that are paleo compliant and keto? Yes, you can have your brownie and eat it too.

1 cup (96 g) almond flour

¾ cup (180 ml) sweetener of choice

½ cup (60 g) unsweetened cocoa powder

½ teaspoon baking powder (¼ teaspoon baking soda + ¼ teaspoon cream of tartar)

¼ teaspoon sea salt

3 large eggs

⅓ cup (80 g) ghee, melted

3 tablespoons (45 ml) water

½ teaspoon pure vanilla extract

⅓ cup (58 g) dark chocolate chips (the darker the better)

½ teaspoon coarse sea salt

Preheat the oven to 350°F (180°C or gas mark 4). Coat an 8 by 8-inch (20 by 20 cm) baking pan with olive oil or cooking spray.

In a medium bowl, whisk together the almond flour, sweetener of choice, cocoa powder, baking powder, and salt.

In a large bowl, whisk together the eggs, ghee, water, and vanilla.

Use a rubber spatula to fold the dry ingredients into the wet ingredients in ¼-cup (30 g) increments. This is to make sure it blends nicely together.

Use the spatula to scrape the sides of the bowl and transfer the batter evenly to the prepared baking dish.

Bake until the desired doneness, 20 to 25 minutes. I usually bake mine for 21 minutes for a gooey texture. If you like your brownies firmer, I suggest baking for 24 minutes.

Allow to cool completely before cutting.

Melt the chocolate chips in the microwave in 30-second increments, stirring in between. Drizzle with a spoon over the brownies and sprinkle with the coarse salt.

Store any extras in an airtight container for up to 1 week.

Peach Crisp

If you're feeling peachy and need a sweet treat, you'll love this recipe. I combine fresh peach slices with all-natural sweeteners and bake it topped with a nutty crumble. Add a dollop of creamy vanilla ice cream, and this fresh recipe is sure to make you smile.

FILLING

6 peaches, sliced (skin on)

⅓ cup (80 ml) pure maple syrup

2 tablespoons (20 g) coconut sugar

1 tablespoon (20 g) honey

1 tablespoon (6 g) tapioca flour

1 teaspoon lemon juice

½ teaspoon pure vanilla extract

TOPPING

½ cup (75 g) pecans or walnuts

¼ cup (24 g) almond flour

2 tablespoons (40 g) honey

2 tablespoons (28 g) ghee or coconut oil, melted

1 tablespoon (6 g) tapioca flour

1 teaspoon lemon zest

¼ teaspoon sea salt

Paleo-friendly vanilla ice cream, for serving (optional)

Filling

Preheat the oven to 350°F (180°C or gas mark 4). Grease a cast-iron skillet or 9 by 9-inch (23 by 23 cm) baking dish of choice.

In a large bowl, combine the peaches, maple syrup, coconut sugar, honey, tapioca flour, lemon juice, and vanilla. Mix together with a spoon until well combined.

Transfer the filling to the prepared baking vessel.

Topping

Add the pecans, almond flour, honey, ghee, tapioca flour, lemon zest, and salt to a food processor. Pulse until the mixture is crumbly.

Evenly top the peach filling with the crumble topping.

Bake until the top is golden and the filling is bubbling, 18 to 20 minutes.

Serve hot with a scoop of ice cream, if desired.

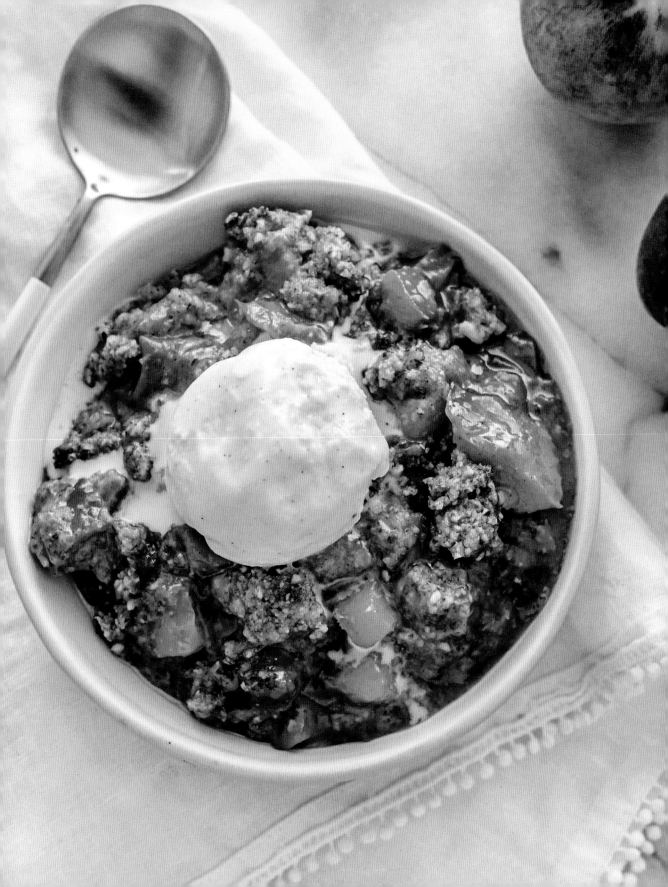

Strawberry Lemonade Bars

YIELD: 9 TO 12 BARS

Refresh your senses with these frozen strawberry lemonade bars. The chewy, nutty crust topped with a creamy strawberry-lemon filling is great for social gatherings or as a weekend treat for the entire family.

CRUST

¾ cup (135 g) pitted Medjool dates

¾ cup (105 g) almonds

¼ cup (35 g) pecans

¼ cup (20 g) unsweetened shredded coconut

Juice of 1 lemon

1 tablespoon (15 ml) pure maple syrup

1 teaspoon lemon zest

½ teaspoon pure vanilla extract

FILLING

1 can (13.5 ounces [378 g]) unsweetened coconut milk, chilled

½ cup (75 g) fresh or frozen strawberries

3½ tablespoons (70 g) honey or sweetener of choice

Juice of 1 lemon

2 tablespoons (12 g) tapioca flour

1 tablespoon (14 g) soft coconut oil

1 teaspoon pure vanilla extract

Zest of ½ lemon

Crust

Line an 8 by 8-inch (20 by 20 cm) baking dish with parchment paper.

Add the dates, almonds, pecans, coconut, lemon juice, maple syrup, lemon zest, and vanilla to a food processor. Pulse until it resembles a crumbly crust.

Transfer the crust to the baking dish and spread out evenly by pressing down to form the crust on top of the parchment paper.

Put the baking dish in the freezer for 10 minutes.

Filling

Add the coconut milk, strawberries, honey, lemon juice, tapioca flour, coconut oil, vanilla, and lemon zest to a blender. Blend on high speed until smooth.

Remove the baking dish from the freezer and pour the filling over the top.

Return the dish to the freezer until the bars harden, at least 3 to 4 hours.

Remove from the freezer and thaw a little before cutting into bars as desired.

Lemon Blueberry Cookies

YIELD: 12 TO 14 COOKIES

This is the perfect cookie for when your cookie monster mood strikes. It's light and lemony and just sweet enough.

COOKIES

2 cups (192 g) almond flour

3 tablespoons (18 g) coconut flour

½ teaspoon baking soda + ½ teaspoon cream of tartar

¼ teaspoon sea salt

1 large egg

½ cup (120 g) coconut oil, melted

½ cup (120 ml) pure maple syrup

2 tablespoons (30 ml) lemon juice

1 teaspoon lemon extract

1 teaspoon lemon zest, plus more for garnish

½ teaspoon pure vanilla extract

½ cup (75 g) blueberries

GLAZE

2 tablespoons (28 g) coconut butter

½ cup (120 ml) coconut cream

2½ tablespoons (37 ml) monk fruit syrup or maple syrup

2 teaspoons lemon juice

½ teaspoon lemon zest

Cookies

Preheat the oven to 350°F (180°C or gas mark 4) and line a baking sheet with parchment paper.

In a medium bowl, whisk together the almond flour, coconut flour, baking powder, and salt.

In a large bowl, whisk together the egg, coconut oil, maple syrup, lemon juice, lemon extract, lemon zest, and vanilla.

Add the dry ingredients to the wet ingredients and mix until completely combined. Fold in the blueberries.

Form the dough into golf ball–size balls and place on the prepared baking sheet, making sure to space them a few inches apart. Gently press down on each ball with the palm of your hand until about 1½ inches (3.8 cm) in diameter.

Bake the cookies until browned around the edges and the center is set, 12 to 15 minutes.

Remove the cookies from the oven and transfer to a rack to cool completely.

Drizzle the cookies with the glaze and sprinkle with the fresh lemon zest.

Store in an airtight container for up to 2 weeks. You can also freeze in an airtight container for up to 3 months.

Glaze

Add all the ingredients to a sauce pan. Bring to a boil and then lower the heat and allow to simmer for 5 minutes, stirring occasionally.

Transfer the glaze to a small bowl and place in the fridge for 5–10 minutes. The glaze will thicken as it cools.

Cinnamon Bun Energy Bites

YIELD: 12 BALLS

These healthy, yet crave-worthy, cinnamon bun-flavored nut balls are perfect for mid-morning or afternoon snacking to help get you over the slump. They'll keep you feeling full and energized for hours.

2 cups walnuts or pecans

⅓ cup chopped dates (around 8 whole dates)

¼ cup almond flour

3 tablespoons maple syrup

1 tablespoon ghee or coconut oil, melted

1½ teaspoons ground cinnamon

¼ teaspoon nutmeg

1 teaspoon pure vanilla

Pinch of salt

COATING

2 tablespoons coconut flour

1¾ tablespoons coconut sugar

¾ teaspoon ground cinnamon

Line a baking sheet with parchment paper.

In a large food processor, pulse the pecans or walnuts until crumbly.

Add the dates, almond flour, maple syrup, ghee or coconut oil, cinnamon, vanilla, and salt. Blend together until it reaches a dough-like consistency. Add more maple syrup or almond flour if needed.

In a separate small bowl, add all the coating ingredients and combine.

Use a small ice cream scoop to form balls the size of golf ball and roll in the coating and place on the baking sheet.

Refrigerate for at least 1 hour before serving or enjoy at room temperature. Store in a glass container in the fridge for up to 1 week.

Paleo Banana Bread

YIELD: 10 TO 12 SERVINGS

This perfect paleo banana bread is moist and filling. If you are looking for a special morning treat to enjoy with your cup of black coffee, look no further.

2 cups (192 g) almond flour

½ cup (48 g) coconut flour

⅓ cup (80 ml) monk fruit or sweetener of choice

2 teaspoons paleo baking powder (1 teaspoon baking soda + 1 teaspoon cream of tartar)

1 teaspoon ground cinnamon

Pinch of sea salt

3 brown or very ripe bananas, peeled and smashed

3 large eggs

3 tablespoons (42 g) coconut oil or ghee, melted

1½ teaspoons pure vanilla extract

1 banana, sliced, of preferred ripeness, for top

Preheat the oven to 350°F (180°C or gas mark 4) and line an 8 by 5-inch (20 by 12.5 cm) loaf pan with parchment paper.

In a medium bowl, whisk together the almond flour, coconut flour, monk fruit, baking powder, cinnamon, and salt.

In a large bowl, whisk together the bananas, eggs, coconut oil, and vanilla.

Carefully fold the dry ingredients into the wet ingredients until combined.

Pour the batter into the prepared loaf pan and top with banana slices. Bake until the top is golden brown and the middle is set, 50 to 60 minutes.

Allow to cool before slicing. Store in an airtight container for up to 2 weeks. Can also be frozen in an airtight container for up to 3 months.

Frozen Fruit Whip

YIELD: 4 SERVINGS

This frozen paleo fruit whip serves as a refreshing and fruity soft serve dessert. Enjoy during those hot summer months or just as an afternoon treat.

1 pound (454 g) frozen fruit of choice

¾ cup (180 ml) unsweetened coconut or almond milk (coconut milk will provide a creamier whip)

¼ cup (60 ml) no-sugar-added pineapple juice

1 teaspoon lemon juice

½ teaspoon pure vanilla extract

1 tablespoon (20 g) honey or sweetener of choice (optional)

Add the frozen fruit, almond milk, pineapple juice, lemon juice, and vanilla to a high-speed blender and blend until it becomes a sorbet consistency. To get the desired consistency, you may need to add more milk.

Taste it and add the honey, if desired, for additional sweetness.

Serve immediately or store in the freezer for later enjoyment.

Note

Store in a freezer-safe container for up to 3 months. Before serving, set the container out at room temperature for 10 minutes. Add the frozen mixture to a blender and rewhip.

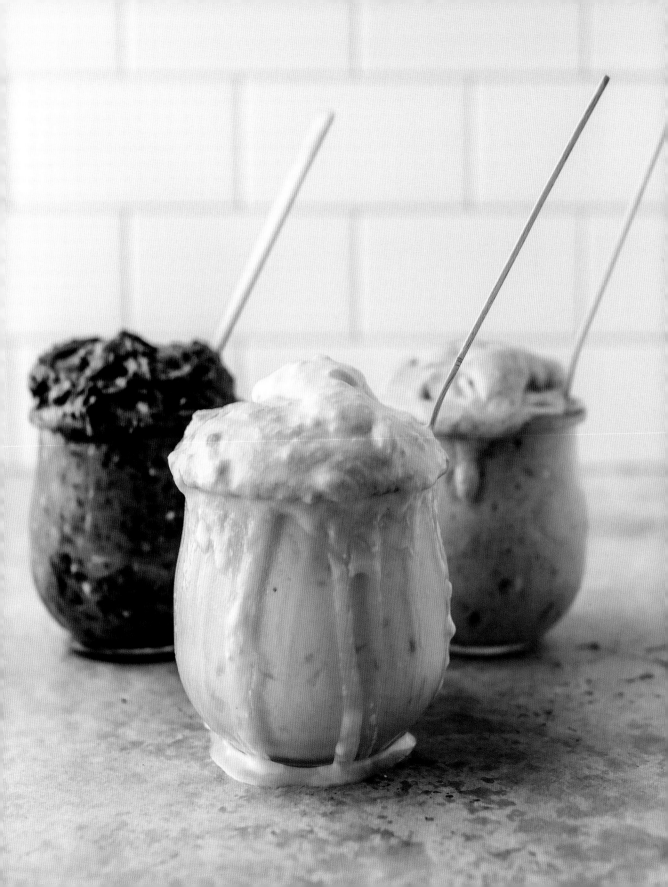

No-Fuss Fudgy Brownies

YIELD: 9 SERVINGS

So fudgy, dense, and perfectly soft, these brownies are made with paleo baking flour, which is a premade blend of almond flour, coconut flour, and starches. For sweetness (because these are definitely sweet), we use coconut sugar and maple syrup. Want more good news? You don't need to break out your stand mixer. This dessert really is easy!

PALEO SIMPLE

1 cup (144 g) coconut sugar

½ cup (120 ml) pure maple syrup

¼ cup (56 g) coconut oil, melted

¼ cup (56 g) ghee, melted

2 large eggs

1½ teaspoons vanilla extract

¾ cups (69 g) paleo baking flour

¼ cup (20 g) unsweetened cacao or cocoa powder

Preheat the oven to 400°F (200°C, or gas mark 6). Line a 9 x 9-inch (23 x 23 cm) baking pan with parchment paper.

In a large bowl, stir together the coconut sugar, maple syrup, oil, and ghee until well combined.

Add the eggs and vanilla. Stir well.

Stir in the paleo baking flour and cacao powder until well combined. Transfer the batter to the prepared pan.

Bake for 17 to 20 minutes or until a toothpick inserted into the center of the brownies comes out with crumbs. The toothpick should not be clean but it shouldn't be completely wet either. (You're going to be on the lower side of that time if using metal and on the higher side of that time if using glass or ceramic.)

After baking, cool until set, about 15 minutes, on the counter or a wire rack. Remove the brownies from the pan by lifting the edges of the parchment paper and slice into 9 squares.

Note

As a general rule, light-colored metal pans are favored for brownies because they cook evenly and prevent over-browning. You can (and I have) use glass or ceramic, but be aware that this type of cooking vessel means your batter may need to cook a bit longer. Since it takes longer for the center to cook, it's also easier to burn the edge pieces, so keep a close eye on it.

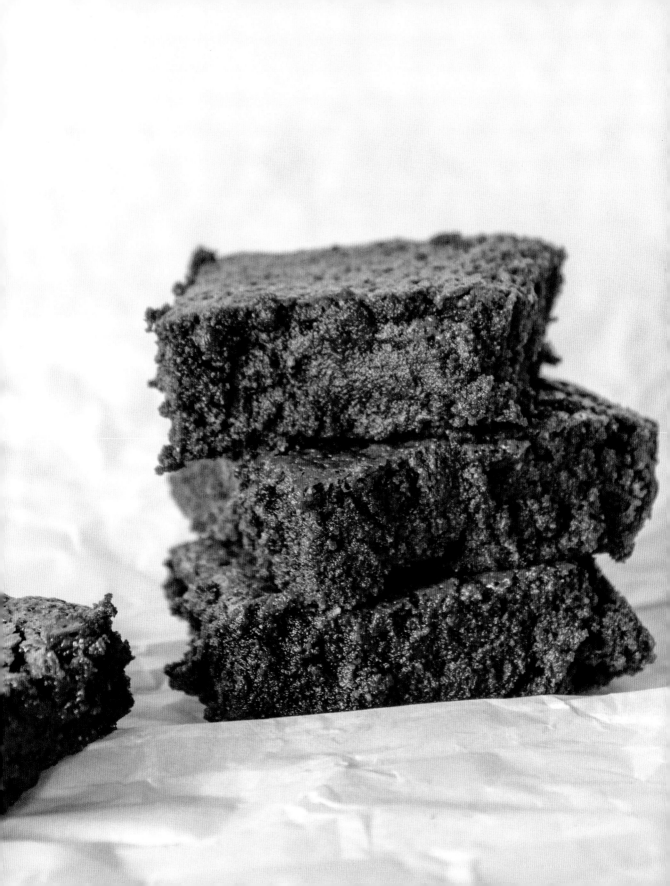

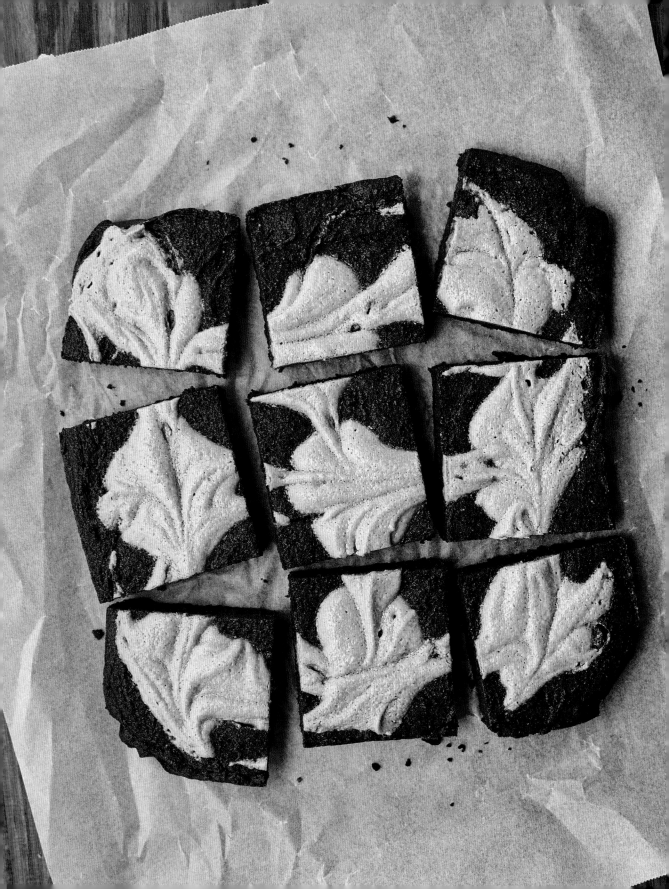

Cashew Butter Swirl Brownies

YIELD: 12 BROWNIES

These brownies are super fudgy and have a sweet swirl of cashew butter on top. They are pretty, but they taste even better than they look.

BROWNIES

⅔ cup (128 g) coconut sugar

½ cup (120 ml) melted butter-flavored coconut oil

3 large eggs, at room temperature

1 teaspoon vanilla extract

½ cup (56 g) almond flour

⅓ cup (27 g) cacao powder

2 tablespoons (15 g) coconut flour

¼ teaspoon salt

2 tablespoons (30 ml) water

CASHEW BUTTER SWIRL

½ cup (120 g) cashew butter

2 tablespoons (30 ml) maple syrup

1 tablespoon (15 ml) melted coconut oil

Preheat the oven to 350°F (180°C or gas mark 4). Line a 9 by 9-inch (23 by 23 cm) baking pan with parchment paper.

Make the brownies: Combine the coconut sugar, coconut oil, eggs, and vanilla in a large bowl. Stir until well combined. Add the almond flour, cacao powder, coconut flour, salt, and water and stir until no dry spots remain. Scoop into the prepared pan and spread evenly.

Make the swirl: Combine the cashew butter, maple syrup, and coconut oil in a small bowl. Stir until smooth. Drop spoonfuls of the mixture on top of the brownies and use a butter knife to swirl the cashew butter with the brownie mixture. Swirl the knife back and forth or in circles.

Bake for 20 minutes, or until set.

Let cool, and then cut and serve.

Store leftovers, covered, in the refrigerator for up to a week.

Strawberry Mini Cheesecakes

YIELD: 10 SERVINGS

Cheesecake with no dairy is possible. The lemon juice gives it the tang that usually comes from the cream cheese. This dessert is no-bake, not too sweet, and so heavenly. You'll need to soak the cashews for 4 hours ahead of time, but if you are in a hurry, soak the cashews in hot water for 1 hour; change the water a couple times as it cools.

CRUST

1 cup (116 g) raw almonds

1 cup (135 g) pitted dates

¼ teaspoon salt

1 tablespoon (15 ml) lemon juice

CHEESECAKE

2 cups (290 g) raw cashews, soaked in water for at least 4 hours

¼ cup (60 ml) melted coconut oil

3 tablespoons (45 ml) maple syrup

1 tablespoon (15 ml) lemon juice

½ teaspoon salt

1 teaspoon vanilla extract

8 ounces (227 g) strawberries, stemmed and sliced

Line a muffin tin with 10 parchment liners.

Make the crust: Place the almonds, dates, salt, and lemon juice in a food processor or high-powered blender. Process until the mixture is combined. It should stick together easily and the almonds should be broken down.

Divide the mixture among the 10 muffin liners and press down into crusts. Place in the refrigerator while you make the cheesecake.

Make the cheesecake: Drain the cashews and rinse with water. Place the cashews in a high-powdered blender. Add the coconut oil, maple syrup, lemon juice, salt, and vanilla. Blend on high speed until smooth. Add the strawberries and blend again until no pieces remain.

Remove the muffin tin from the refrigerator and pour the cheesecake filling on top of each crust. Place in the refrigerator for at least 2 hours to chill, or in the freezer for firmer cheesecakes.

Once firm, remove the cheesecakes from the tin and serve.

Store leftovers, covered, in the refrigerator for up to 10 days or freeze for up to 3 months.

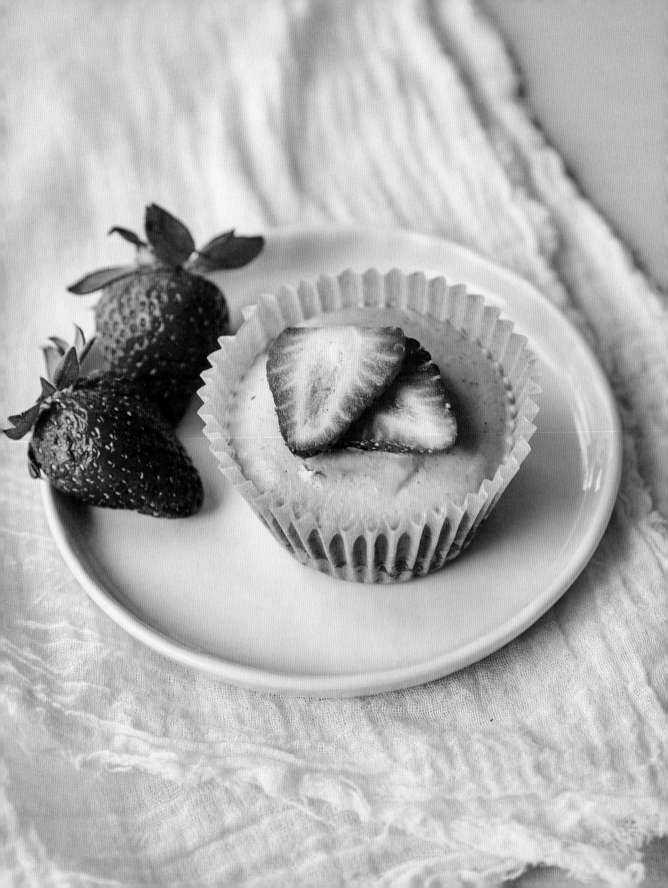

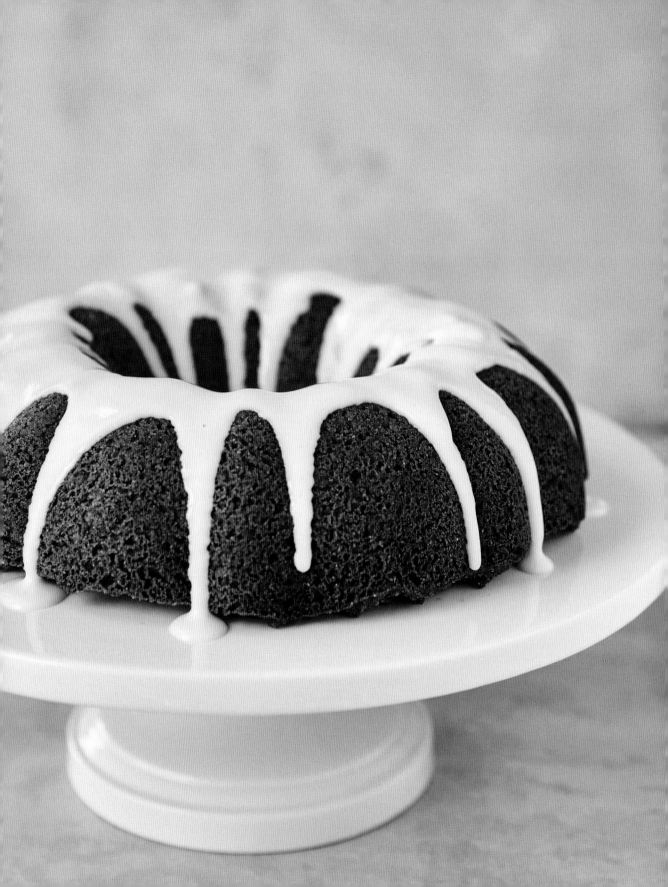

Lemon Poppy Seed Bundt Cake

YIELD: 8 TO 10 SERVINGS

This cake is moist, tender, and sweet. Topped with a simple and bright glaze, it is fancy enough for a special occasion and easy enough to whip up anytime.

CAKE

3 cups (336 g) almond flour

⅓ cup (40 g) coconut flour

3 tablespoons (29 g) poppy seeds

2 teaspoons (10 g) baking soda

¾ teaspoon salt

½ cup (120 g) ghee

⅔ cup (128 g) coconut sugar

3 large eggs, at room temperature

Zest of 2 lemons

½ cup (120 ml) lemon juice (from 3 lemons)

¼ cup (60 ml) water

GLAZE

¼ cup (60 g) coconut butter/manna

1 tablespoon (15 ml) maple syrup

2 tablespoons (30 ml) lemon juice

⅛ teaspoon salt

1 teaspoon vanilla extract

Preheat the oven to 325°F (170°C or gas mark 3). Grease a 12-cup (3 L) Bundt pan very well with coconut oil or ghee.

Make the cake: Combine the almond flour, coconut flour, poppy seeds, baking soda, and salt in a medium-size bowl.

Combine the ghee and coconut sugar in a large bowl. Cream with a hand mixer. Add the eggs and mix again until smooth. Add the lemon zest, juice, and water and mix again.

Add in the dry mixture and mix well, until no dry spots remain.

Pour into the prepared pan and bake for 45 minutes, or until set. Let cool for 30 minutes and then remove from the pan. I always have good luck carefully loosening it first with a butter knife along the sides. Place a large plate on top of the pan and flip it over to release the cake.

Make the glaze: If the coconut butter is very hard, place it in the microwave for 30 seconds and stir well to combine. Combine the coconut butter, maple syrup, lemon juice, salt, and vanilla in a small bowl. Mix well and drizzle on top of the cake. Slice and serve.

Store leftovers, covered, at room temperature for 2 days, or refrigerated for longer.

Banoffee Pie

YIELD: 6 TO 8 SERVINGS

This banana toffee pie is incredibly rich. It's a no-bake dessert that has a sweet caramel layer topped with thick banana slices and a mountain of billowy coconut whipped cream.

CRUST

2 cups (299 g) raw sunflower seeds

1 cup (135 g) pitted dates

¼ teaspoon salt

2–3 tablespoons (30–45 ml) water

CARAMEL

1 cup (135 g) pitted dates

½ cup (128 g) sunflower seed butter, such as SunButter

¼ teaspoon salt

2 teaspoons (10 ml) vanilla extract

3–4 tablespoons (45–60 ml) water

PIE

3 bananas, sliced into ¼-inch (6 mm) slices

1–2 tablespoons (15–30 ml) lemon juice

9 ounces (255 g) coconut whipped topping

1 ounce (28 g) dairy-free chocolate, shaved (optional)

Line a deep-dish pie pan with parchment paper.

Make the crust: Combine the sunflower seeds, dates, and salt in a food processor and blend until mostly combined. Add the water, starting with 2 tablespoons (30 ml) and adding the rest if needed. The mixture should hold together, but it will be sticky. Press into the bottom and up the sides of the pie plate. Place in the refrigerator while you make the caramel.

Make the caramel: Combine the dates, sunflower seed butter, salt, and vanilla in a food processor. Add the water, starting with 3 tablespoons (45 ml) and adding the rest if needed, and blend until smooth. Scoop the mixture on top of the crust and smooth evenly. (If making ahead, stop at this step, cover, and refrigerate.)

Make the pie: Place the bananas in a medium-size bowl and add the lemon juice. Gently toss to cover all the banana slices. Evenly arrange the bananas on top of the caramel.

Top with the coconut whipped topping and serve immediately, or place in the refrigerator until serving. Dust with the shaved chocolate before serving, if desired.

This pie is best served the same day, but it can be stored, covered, in the refrigerator for up to 3 days.

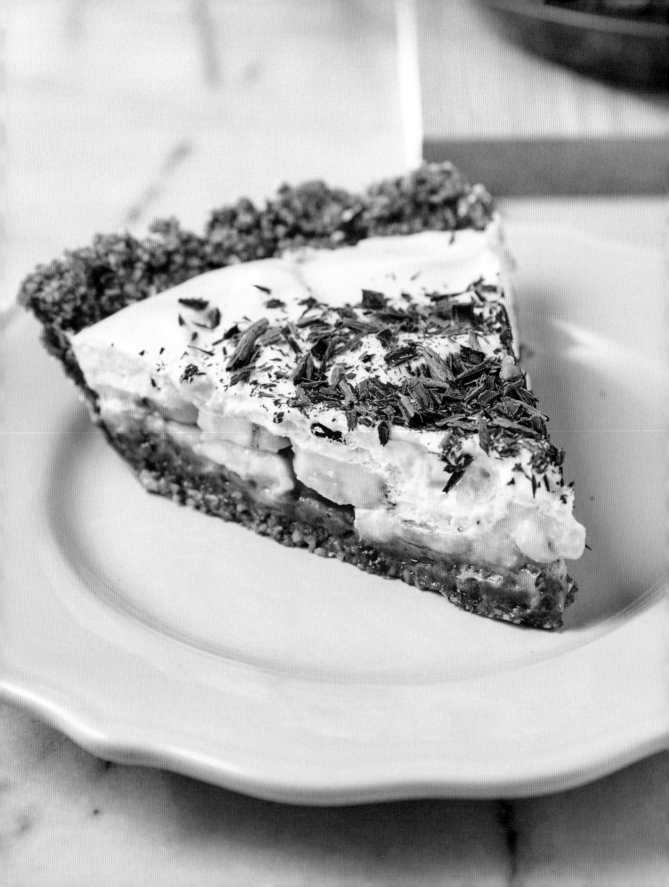

Banana Blondies

YIELD: 12 BLONDIES

I love making banana bread, but sometimes I want a different treat with the ripe bananas needing to be used. These thick, moist bars are sweet and soft and taste similar to banana bread, but in bar form. The frosting makes them extra delicious.

BLONDIES

2 cups (224 g) almond flour

¼ cup (30 g) coconut flour

½ cup (96 g) coconut sugar

½ teaspoon salt

1½ teaspoons (4 g) ground cinnamon

½ cup (120 ml) almond milk

1 cup (240 ml) pureed banana (2½–3 medium bananas)

FROSTING

¼ cup (62 g) coconut butter/manna

¼ cup (60 ml) maple syrup

⅛ teaspoon salt

1 teaspoon vanilla extract

2 tablespoons (26 g) butter-flavored coconut oil

Preheat the oven to 350°F (180°C or gas mark 4). Line a 9 by 9-inch (23 by 23 cm) pan with parchment paper or grease well with coconut oil.

Make the blondies: Combine the almond flour, coconut flour, coconut sugar, salt, and cinnamon in a large bowl and stir well. Add the almond milk and banana and mix until no dry spots remain. The mixture will be thick. Scoop into the prepared pan and bake for 35–40 minutes, or until set. Let cool before frosting.

Make the frosting: Combine the coconut butter, maple syrup, salt, vanilla, and coconut oil in a small bowl. Stir until well mixed and smooth. Spread over the blondies and place in the refrigerator to chill.

Slice and serve.

Store leftovers, covered, in the refrigerator for up to a week.

Citrus Snack Cake

YIELD: 8 SERVINGS

The combination of orange and lemon in this cake is wonderfully refreshing. It is simple to make and moist—a nice, light treat.

3 cups (336 g) almond flour

¾ cup (108 g) maple sugar or (144 g) coconut sugar

¼ cup (30 g) coconut flour

1 teaspoon baking soda

¼ teaspoon salt

Zest of 1 orange

Zest of 1 lemon

3 large eggs, at room temperature

½ cup (120 ml) melted ghee or butter-flavored coconut oil

¼ cup (60 ml) lemon juice

¼ cup (60 ml) orange juice

1 teaspoon vanilla extract

Preheat the oven to 325°F (170°C or gas mark 3). Line a 9-inch (23 cm) round pan with parchment paper or grease well with coconut oil.

Combine the almond flour, maple sugar, coconut flour, baking soda, and salt in a large bowl. Mix well.

Add the orange and lemon zests, eggs, ghee, lemon and orange juices, and vanilla. Stir well, until everything is mixed and no dry spots remain.

Pour into the prepared pan and bake for 35 minutes, or until set.

Let cool, then slice and serve warm. This is also great cold from the fridge.

Store leftovers, covered, in the refrigerator for up to a week.

Butternut Squash Pecan Crumble

YIELD: 6 SERVINGS

I don't tolerate pumpkin well, but I wanted a pumpkin-like dessert and this turned out better than I planned. It's a smooth, creamy layer of squash topped with the best-ever crumb topping. I served this at my family Thanksgiving and it was a huge hit. It will definitely become a yearly tradition.

SQUASH FILLING

1 butternut squash (about 3½ pounds [1.6 kg])

2 tablespoons (30 g) ghee

2 tablespoons (30 ml) maple syrup

2 large eggs

½ teaspoon salt

1 teaspoon ground cinnamon

1 teaspoon pumpkin pie spice

¼ cup (30 g) coconut flour

TOPPING

1½ cups (168 g) finely chopped raw pecans

¼ cup (30 g) coconut flour

3 tablespoons (40 g) ghee, at room temperature

1 teaspoon ground cinnamon

2 tablespoons (30 ml) maple syrup

¼ teaspoon salt

Preheat the oven to 425°F (220°C or gas mark 7). Line a baking sheet with parchment paper. Line a 9 by 9-inch (23 by 23 cm) pan with parchment paper or grease well with coconut oil.

Make the squash filling: Cut the butternut squash lengthwise and scoop out the seeds. Place cut side down on the prepared baking sheet and bake for 50–55 minutes, or until tender. Let cool for about 15 minutes, or until easily handled but still warm. Decrease the heat to 350°F (180°C or gas mark 4).

Scoop the squash into a large bowl. Add the ghee, maple syrup, eggs, salt, cinnamon, pumpkin pie spice, and coconut flour. Stir well, mashing any chunks. Use an immersion blender if you want it really smooth.

Scoop the butternut squash mixture into the prepared pan.

Make the topping: Combine the pecans, coconut flour, ghee, cinnamon, maple syrup, and salt in a medium-size bowl. Mix until combined and crumbly. Evenly sprinkle the mixture on top of the squash.

Bake for 30 minutes, or until the top is lightly brown.

Let cool, then slice and serve.

Store leftovers, covered, in the refrigerator for up to a week.

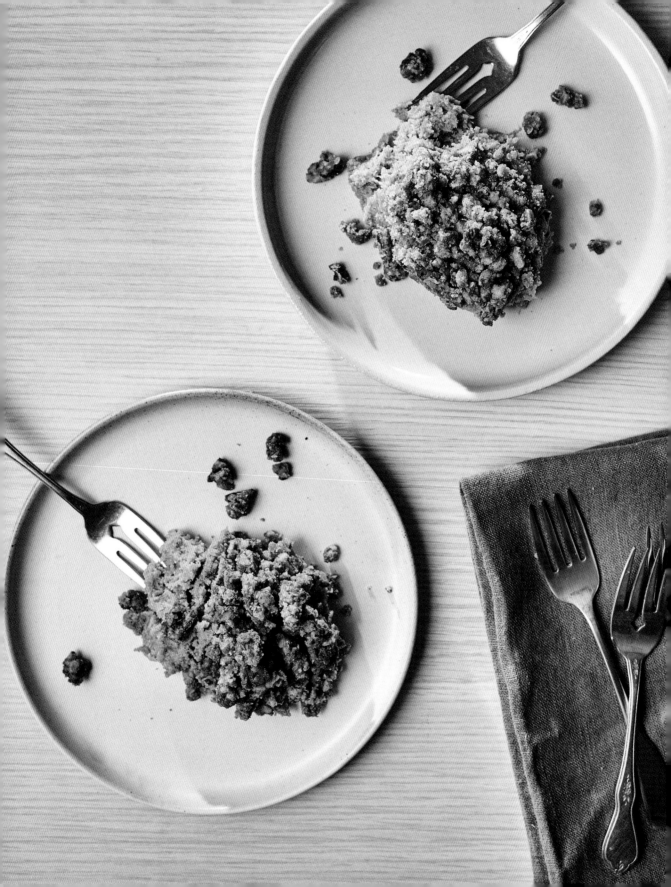

Peppermint Patties

What's better than a creamy cool peppermint center encased by sweet dark chocolate? One that's simple to make. These also make a great gift, because they don't need to be kept in the refrigerator.

¾ cup (186 g) coconut butter/manna

¼ cup (60 ml) melted coconut oil

3–4 tablespoons (45–60 ml) maple syrup

⅛ teaspoon salt

1½ teaspoons (7 ml) peppermint extract

1 cup (180 g) dairy-free chocolate chips

Make sure the coconut butter is soft. If it's hard, warm briefly in the microwave and stir well. Line a baking sheet with parchment or wax paper.

Combine the coconut butter, coconut oil, maple syrup, salt, and peppermint extract in a small bowl. Mix well. Refrigerate for 10 minutes to firm up.

Roll into 1½-teaspoon balls and press into 1½-inch (4 cm) circles, forming patties. Place on the prepared baking sheet. Repeat with the remaining mixture; it should make 16 total.

Place in the refrigerator for 2 hours to chill.

Melt the chocolate chips in the microwave, stirring every 30 seconds, for about 1½ minutes, or until smooth. Alternatively, melt the chocolate in a small saucepan over low heat, stirring the whole time.

Dip the patties in the melted chocolate, letting the excess drip off, and place back on the baking sheet. Dip all of them and then place in the refrigerator to set.

Once set, they do not need to be refrigerated. Store leftovers, covered, at room temperature for up to a week.

Chocolate Mint Cookies

YIELD: 12 COOKIES

These cookies are mixed completely in the food processor, so they come together quickly. They are slightly crisp on the outside and the inside is fudgy.

1 cup (116 g) raw almonds

1 cup (135 g) pitted dates

2 tablespoons (30 g) almond butter

½ teaspoon salt

¼ cup (20 g) cacao powder

¼ teaspoon baking soda

1 large egg

½ teaspoon peppermint extract

Preheat the oven to 350°F (180°C or gas mark 4). Line a baking sheet with parchment paper.

Blend the almonds in a food processor until fine like flour. Add the dates and almond butter, and blend until it forms a sticky dough. Add the salt, cacao powder, baking soda, and egg and blend again until combined. Add the peppermint extract and blend again.

Scoop into heaping tablespoon (15 g) portions, roll into balls, and place on the prepared baking sheet. Press down slightly and bake for 10–12 minutes. Serve warm, at room temperature, or chilled.

Store leftovers, covered, in the refrigerator for up to 10 days.

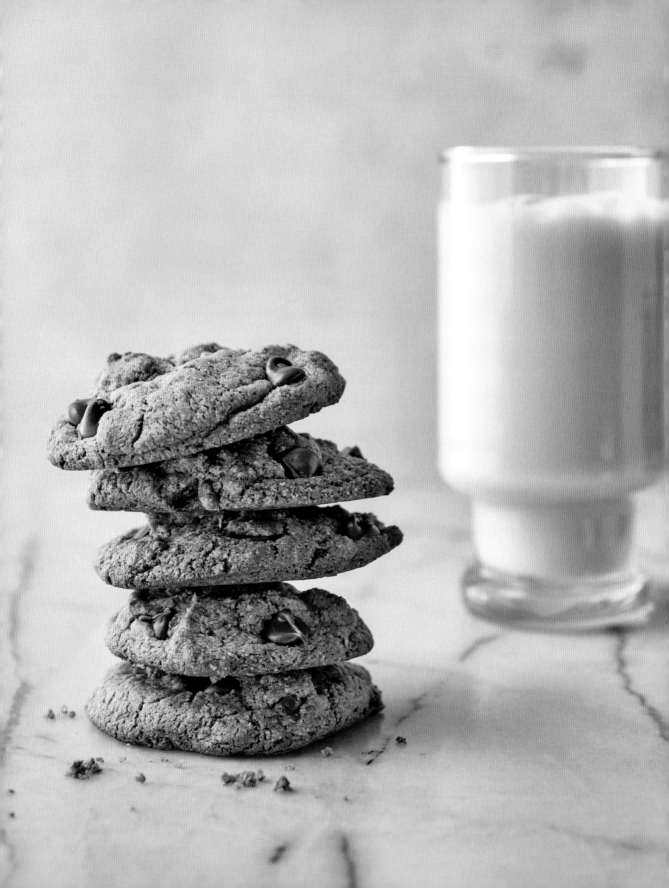

Mike's Favorite Chocolate Chip Cookies

YIELD: 18 COOKIES

Mike is a close family friend who helps me test recipes. These are his absolute favorite. At first he couldn't believe they were paleo, because they taste so much like the originals. If you are in search of the best chocolate chip cookie, this is it!

6 tablespoons (90 g) ghee, at room temperature

¾ cup (144 g) coconut sugar

1 large egg, at room temperature

⅓ cup (80 g) cashew butter

1¼ cups (140 g) almond flour

3 tablespoons (23 g) coconut flour

1 teaspoon vanilla extract

¼ teaspoon salt

1 teaspoon baking soda

1 cup (180 g) dairy-free chocolate chips

Preheat the oven to 350°F (180°C or gas mark 4). Line a baking sheet with parchment paper.

Combine the ghee and coconut sugar in a large bowl. Mix until well combined. A hand mixer works best for this. Add the egg and cashew butter and mix again until smooth. Add the almond flour, coconut flour, vanilla, salt, and baking soda and mix until no dry spots remain. Fold in the chocolate chips (keep some aside if you want to add more in step 3).

Scoop the mixture into heaping tablespoon (15 g) portions and roll into balls. Place them on the prepared baking sheet and press down just slightly. Add a couple more chocolate chips on top of each one, if desired.

Bake for 10–12 minutes, or until the edges look done. The center will still look soft. Let cool for at least 10 minutes before removing from the pan. They are soft when they first come out, but will firm up as they cool. They are great served warm.

Store leftovers, covered, at room temperature for up to 2 days or in the refrigerator for up to 10 days.

Thick Sugar Cookies

These cookies are soft and sweet—the perfect cookies. They're an incredible remake of the classic that is so well loved. Maple sugar is lighter than coconut sugar, making cookies that look more like traditional sugar cookies. Coconut sugar works great as well, but the cookies will be slightly darker.

1⅔ cups (187 g) almond flour

3 tablespoons (23 g) coconut flour

½ teaspoon baking soda

¼ teaspoon salt

½ cup (120 g) ghee or (104 g) butter-flavored coconut oil, at room temperature

½ cup (72 g) maple sugar or (96 g) coconut sugar

1 large egg, at room temperature

1 teaspoon vanilla extract

Preheat the oven to 325°F (170°C or gas mark 3). Line a baking sheet with parchment paper.

Combine the almond flour, coconut flour, baking soda, and salt in a medium-size bowl. Stir well.

Combine the ghee and maple sugar in a large bowl. Mix with a hand mixer until combined. Add the egg and vanilla and mix again until smooth.

Add the dry ingredients to the wet ingredients and mix again until fully combined, with no dry spots remaining.

Scoop into 1 tablespoon (15 g) portions, roll into balls, and place on the prepared baking sheet. Press down slightly and bake for 10–12 minutes. Serve warm or at room temperature.

Store leftovers, covered, in the refrigerator for up to 10 days.

Classic Chocolate Fudge

YIELD: 10 TO 12 SERVINGS

This fudge makes a great gift, because it doesn't need to be kept in the refrigerator to stay firm. Making the homemade sweetened condensed milk takes a little time, but it's very easy. If you're looking for a fudge you can give or set out at parties, this is it!

One 13.5-ounce (378 ml) can full-fat coconut milk

⅓ cup (80 ml) maple syrup

⅛ teaspoon salt

2½ cups (450 g) unsweetened chocolate chips

1 teaspoon vanilla extract

Line a loaf pan with parchment paper or grease well with coconut oil.

Combine the coconut milk, maple syrup, and salt in a 2-quart (2 L) saucepan over medium heat and whisk until the mixture is boiling. Decrease the heat to low and simmer until the mixture is thickened, 25–45 minutes, depending on how low your setting goes. It should measure about 1¼ cups (300 ml) when done.

Place the chocolate chips in a large bowl. Pour the coconut milk mixture over the chocolate chips. The heat will melt them. Add the vanilla and stir until completely smooth.

Pour into the prepared pan and place in the refrigerator to set.

Once set, this does not need to be kept in the refrigerator. Slice and serve.

Store leftovers, covered, at room temperature for up to a week.

Avocado Chocolate Pudding

YIELD: 4 SERVINGS

Do you want to try a decadent and delicious treat that's chock-full of nourishing fats? I bet you do. This chocolate pudding is sweetened with coconut sugar and loaded with real cacao powder, sea salt, and yes, real avocados (but you would never know it!). It's such a nice indulgence that will keep you full with all those healthy fats. I like to enjoy it alongside breakfast—or as a dessert, of course. It's great plain, but you can dress it up with cacao nibs, unsweetened coconut flakes, fresh mint, etc.

⅔ cup (130 g) coconut sugar

2 avocados, peeled and pitted

⅔ cup (160 ml) full-fat canned coconut milk

½ cup (50 g) cacao powder

1 teaspoon (5 ml) pure vanilla extract

¼ teaspoon sea salt

2 to 3 tablespoons (30 to 45 ml) avocado oil or coconut oil, melted

In a food processor, pulse the coconut sugar for a few seconds. Add the avocados, coconut milk, cacao, vanilla, and salt. Process for about 1 minute until smooth, creamy, and thick throughout.

Turn the food processor on low and open the shoot. Slowly drizzle in the oil, 1 tablespoon (15 ml) at a time, until the mixture reaches your desired consistency. I like to use 2 ½ to 3 tablespoons (37 to 45 ml).

Store in an airtight container in the refrigerator for up to 5 days.

Cheesecake Dip

YIELD: 2 CUPS (473 ML), ABOUT 10 SERVINGS

Creamy and sweetened just right, this makes a great dip for fruit or grain-free cookies for an indulgent treat. You will need to soak the cashews for 6 hours. If you are short on time, soak them for 1 hour in hot water, changing the water a couple times as it cools.

2 cups (300 g) raw cashews

3 tablespoons (45 ml) maple syrup

½ teaspoon salt

2 tablespoons (30 ml) lemon juice

1 teaspoon vanilla extract

Soak the cashews in water for 6 hours to soften. Drain, rinse the cashews, and place in a high-powered blender.

Add the maple syrup, salt, lemon juice, and vanilla. Blend until smooth, stopping and scraping down the sides as needed. This may take 5–10 minutes; just be patient as you stop and scrape down. It will get smooth and creamy.

Pour into a serving bowl and serve immediately as a dip for fruit or grain-free cookies.

Store leftovers, covered, in the refrigerator for up to 10 days.

Almond Butter Banana Bundt Cake

YIELD: 8 TO 10 SERVINGS

This is a soft and tender cake with a buttery crumb, topped with an incredible caramel-like glaze. It looks fancy but is easy to make.

CAKE

1 cup (225 g) mashed or pureed banana (about 3 medium bananas)

½ cup (96 g) coconut sugar

½ cup (120 g) almond butter

2 large eggs

1 teaspoon vanilla extract

3 cups (336 g) almond flour

¼ cup (30 g) coconut flour

1 teaspoon ground cinnamon

½ teaspoon salt

1 teaspoon baking soda

¾ cup (180 ml) almond milk

GLAZE

¼ cup (60 g) almond butter

¼ cup (60 ml) melted coconut oil

¼ cup (60 ml) maple syrup

1 teaspoon vanilla extract

Preheat the oven to 350°F (180°C or gas mark 4). Grease a 12-cup (3 L) Bundt pan well with coconut oil.

Make the cake: Combine the banana, coconut sugar, almond butter, eggs, and vanilla in a large bowl. Stir well.

In a separate bowl, add the almond flour, coconut flour, cinnamon, salt, and baking soda. Stir to combine. Add the dry ingredients to the wet and stir to combine. Add the almond milk and stir again until no dry spots remain.

Pour the mixture into the prepared Bundt pan and spread evenly. Bake for 40 minutes, or until set.

Let cool for 10 minutes. Remove from the pan. I always have good luck carefully loosening it first with a butter knife along the sides. Place a large plate on top and flip it over.

Make the glaze: Combine the almond butter, coconut oil, maple syrup, and vanilla in a small bowl. Stir until smooth. Drizzle over the cooled cake. Slice and serve.

Store leftovers, covered, in the refrigerator for up to a week.

Index